AF675257

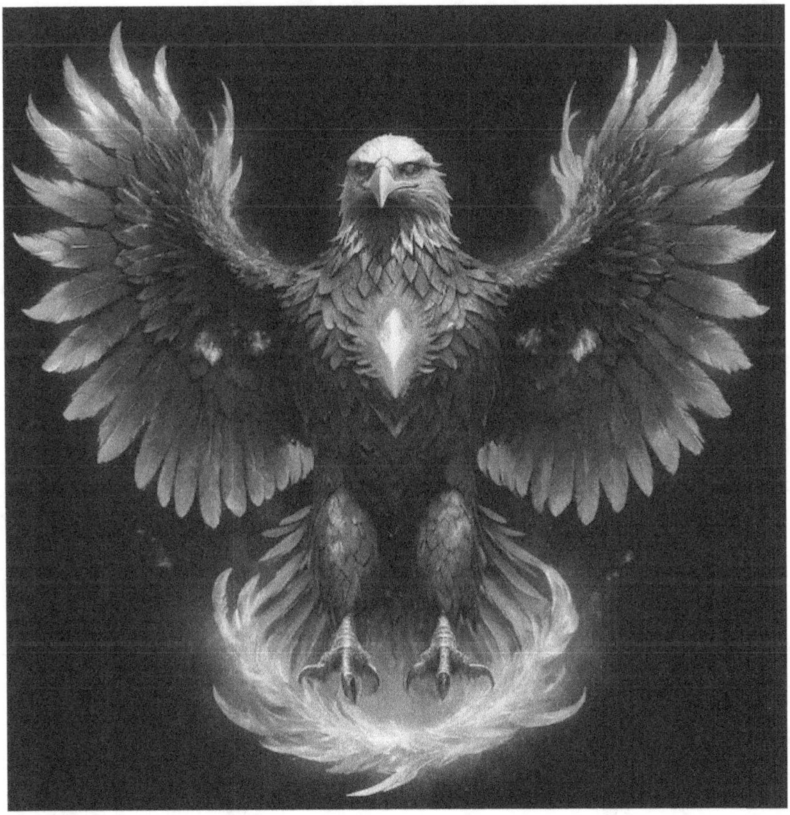

ISBN: [978-81-981246-7-8] MRP - 9849 /-

To the character of a bird :

AUTHOR - CHILDEYE

EDITOR - CHILDEYE

Breathe Until We Can’t

"Part - Three & Four"

SM-27 #sm27

M-41 #m41

#mbook

#childeye

SWANPUBLICA

***Breathe Until We Can't* Series**

Part - 3 "After We Let Go"

In a bar's dim light, shadows flicker,
Where laughter once danced, now thoughts grow thicker,
Jack stares into the glass, a world in disarray,
Haunted by memories that refuse to decay.

The clinking of bottles, a bitter-sweet sound,
In every drop spilled, a past left unbound,
Yet in the chaos, a flicker of grace,
An echo of friendship, a warm, tender space.

With each passing moment, the ghosts come alive,
In the stories they share, in the love that survives,
For though grief may linger, it teaches us well,
To cherish the laughter, the light in the hell.

In the quietest moments, the guilt creeps in,
A weight on her shoulders, a constant chagrin,
Sophie sifts through charts, searching for signs,
Of what she could've changed, in those tangled lines.

The whispers of patients, their stories unfold,
Each breath a reminder of the life they uphold,
Yet Emily lingers, a ghost by her side,
In every heartbeat, her love, her pride.

In therapy's grasp, she wrestles the pain,
Learning that grief isn't something to feign,

With every confession, the burden grows light,
As she finds the strength to embrace the night.

Underneath the humor, the scars run deep,
Jack chuckles at Amelia, but can't help but weep,
For every quip shared holds a shard of his heart,
A reminder of friendship, a life torn apart.

In the chaos of laughter, the pain finds a way,
To weave through the jokes, to darken the day,
Yet within the banter, a flicker ignites,
A hope for the future, a chance for new sights.

As the nights grow longer and the drinks start to flow,
Jack finds a warmth in the love that can grow,
For even in sorrow, in the shadows they tread,
A spark of connection can light up the dread.

In the corridors bright, where breaths intertwine,
Sophie stands vigilant, her heart a soft line,
Each patient a story, a journey to share,
Yet Emily's presence is heavy in the air.

With Oliver's laughter, a reminder of grace,
In each tender moment, she finds her own space,
For hope can rise gently, like dawn from the night,
In the battles we fight, we discover our light.

She gathers her strength, with each patient she holds,
Transforming her sorrow into stories retold,
Through the walk for awareness, she begins to see,
That in every goodbye, there's a chance to be free.

In the heart of the city, where stories collide,
Jack finds himself drifting, lost in the tide,

Yet amid all the chaos, a thread starts to weave,
Connecting the moments, the love we believe.

With Amelia's laughter, he learns how to feel,
The weight of his burdens, he starts to reveal,
In the echo of memories, he finds a way through,
For love's gentle hand can mend what we knew.

Sophie steps forward, her project takes flight,
In the name of remembrance, she chases the light,
For every lost soul holds a lesson so dear,
In honouring their life, we find ways to heal.

Preface

In the tumultuous journey of life, few experiences shape us as profoundly as love and loss. As I pen the pages of Breath Until We Can't : *After We Let Go*, the third installment of this series, I am acutely aware of the delicate balance between grief and healing that each character must navigate. Jack and Sophie, my beloved characters, are both grappling with the weight of their pasts. Jack, once a promising grad student, finds himself adrift in a world where the echoes of laughter and joy have been replaced by solitude and regret because of the depression. His role at The Tipsy Oak, a dimly lit bar, symbolizes the dimming of his once-bright aspirations. Here, amidst the clinking glasses and whispered secrets, he struggles to confront his grief, relying on old friendships and fleeting connections to fill the void left by the loss of his closest friend and his own can-do attitude or spirit. No one knows why one or the other faces depression but that's the reality of our world.

Sophie, on the other hand, embodies the resilience of the human spirit. Working long shifts at St. Luke's Medical Center, she confronts the reality of lung diseases daily—reminders of her friend Emily's tragic battle. The weight of guilt hangs heavily on her shoulders, compounded by the faces of patients who evoke bittersweet memories of love and loss. Her journey through grief therapy reveals not only her vulnerabilities but also the strength required to face the truth of her emotions.

This part of the series delves deeply into the human psyche, exploring the intersections of trauma, guilt, and the quest for meaning amid chaos. Jack's and Sophie's paths converge as they navigate their individual struggles, each grappling with their own forms of helplessness. Their stories reflect the universal challenge of moving forward while carrying the burden of those left behind. As I wrote these chapters, I was reminded of the fragility of life and the importance of embracing vulnerability. Humour often emerges from the shadows of sorrow, a lifeline to remind us that even in our darkest moments, laughter can pierce through the veil of grief.

Ultimately, *After We Let Go* is about the delicate process of healing, the small steps we take toward acceptance, and the power of love that endures despite loss. It is a tribute to those who have shaped our lives and a call to honour their memories by embracing the future.

As you journey through these pages, I invite you to reflect on your own experiences with love and loss. May you find solace in the stories of Jack and Sophie, and may their resilience inspire you to confront your own shadows. Together, let us explore the uncharted waters of grief, healing, and the bonds that transcend even the deepest sorrow.

With care,

INDEX

Chapter 1: Three Years Later

Jack has dropped out of PhD course, unable to find the same sense of purpose he once believed he could. He now works at *The Tipsy Oak,* a small, dimly lit bar that reeks of spilled beer and faded dreams. The bar's atmosphere mirrors Jack's own life—dark, worn out, and full of unspoken regret. Disheveled and disconnected, he barely makes enough to get by, his shifts a monotonous blur of pouring drinks and pretending to care about the regulars' stories. His once carefree attitude has crumbled under the weight of grief and guilt. Financially struggling, Jack's pride keeps him from asking for help, but he's been relying on the kindness of his old college friend, Zach, to let him crash on his couch. Each day, Jack feels himself slipping further away from the person he used to be. At *The Tipsy Oak,* Jack wears a mask of indifference, but late at night, when the bar clears out and he's left alone to close up, he finds himself replaying moments from the past, unable to escape the ghosts of those he's lost. The guitar pick is always in his pocket, a reminder of Liam, but it feels heavier now—a symbol of what could have been and what Jack fears he'll never become.

Jack's physical and mental health has been on a steep decline since he took admission for the PhD. He suffers from chronic insomnia, spending nights tossing and turning, staring at the ceiling while the shadows of his thoughts grow darker. The lack of sleep has taken its toll—his eyes are bloodshot, dark circles permanently etched under them, making him appear older than his years. Despite the constant exhaustion, he can't shut his mind off.

The insomnia is compounded by frequent, debilitating migraines that come in relentless waves. The throbbing in his head feels like a hammer pounding against his skull, leaving him nauseated and sensitive to light. At work, the dim lighting of *The Tipsy Oak* helps mask the pain, but the migraines always linger in the background, making it harder for him to focus.

Jack knows something is wrong, but he refuses to go to a doctor, too stubborn and afraid to face the reality of his deteriorating condition. He brushes off his symptoms, convincing himself it's just stress, that it'll eventually pass. Instead of seeking proper medical treatment, he self-medicates. Over-the-counter painkillers have become his crutch—ibuprofen, aspirin, anything to dull the pain for a while. He takes them more often than he should, popping them without a second thought, even though they do little to truly alleviate his suffering.

In his drawer at Zach's apartment, there's a prescription for strong sleeping pills, prescribed months ago by a concerned physician after Jack's third consecutive sleepless night in the ER. But the bottle remains unfilled. Jack refuses to rely on something so serious—he fears addiction or the loss of control that might come with it. The idea of being dependent on pills terrifies him, just as he saw Liam become reliant on medications in his final days. Despite the growing physical toll, Jack avoids any real medical intervention, afraid of what he might uncover and preferring to numb his pain with makeshift solutions. The migraines are getting worse, though, and the insomnia has become more than just a nuisance—it's shaping his every waking moment, slowly pulling him further into a spiral of self-neglect.

...

Sophie has thrown herself fully into her work at St. Luke's Medical Center, particularly in the respiratory ward, where she spends long hours caring for patients with conditions like COPD, ALS, and other lung diseases. For it she has gained enough experience at the NY-Presbyterian Hospital. Her life now revolves around the endless cycle of diagnosing, treating, and comforting patients struggling with the same diseases that took her best friend, Emily. Each day brings her face-to-face with the cruel realities of these diseases—the slow, painful progression, the mounting exhaustion in patients' eyes, and the overwhelming fear in their families. Despite her passion for the work, there's a part of Sophie that remains emotionally distant, particularly when it comes to Emily's case. She skilfully dodges questions about her personal connection to COPD or ALS. Even when her colleagues bring up similar cases, Sophie remains composed, avoiding any mention of the personal scars that still weigh heavily on her heart. It's as though she's constructed a wall between her professional life and the personal grief she hasn't fully processed.

Her patients admire her calm demeanour, and doctors respect her sharp intuition and dedication. She monitors every patient closely—checking oxygen levels, administering bronchodilators, and coordinating therapies designed to improve lung function, all with a sense of precision that comes from deeply understanding the stakes involved. Her experience working with Dr. Sara Thomspon, Emily's pulmonologist, has honed her skills, and Sophie often participates in clinical rounds and discussions about cutting-edge respiratory treatments. However, beneath the surface, the emotional toll is significant. Each patient with COPD reminds her of Emily. The familiar sound of oxygen tanks, the laboured breathing, and the constant adjustments to therapy feel like echoes of her past. Whenever she's faced with a particularly difficult case, she flashes back to Emily gasping for breath during their protests or collapsing into her arms. But Sophie remains steadfast, never revealing the depth of her personal pain to her patients or colleagues. Her long shifts at the hospital have become a means of escape. She works through the night, often volunteering for the hardest shifts in the respiratory unit. The fatigue of overwork helps dull the sharpness of her grief, and she uses the constant hum of hospital life as a buffer against her personal memories. When she's not on shift, she attends conferences and reads research on ALS and COPD, trying to contribute to the fight against these diseases from every angle.

...

Sophie's day begins early at St. Luke's Medical Center. She arrives before the sun fully rises, her scrubs crisp, but her eyes showing the weight of sleepless nights. Grabbing her tablet, she dives into patient charts before the shift officially begins. Her first task: reviewing each patient's oxygen levels, breathing patterns, and overall respiratory condition. She meticulously notes down any changes—oxygen saturation, the frequency of coughing fits, signs of distress—and flags anything unusual for further examination. She's already mentally organizing treatment plans, knowing the critical importance of catching small changes before they become catastrophic.

Her rounds start with a quick visit to the nurses' station, where she gathers updates on overnight changes. A few patients required increased oxygen support during the night, and one had a severe coughing fit that left him gasping. Sophie makes a mental note to follow up with Dr. Richards on this patient later. But first, she heads into the rooms.

Each interaction feels routine yet urgent. With a practiced smile, she checks on Mr. Diaz, a COPD patient who has been relying on oxygen therapy for months. His oxygen saturation is lower than it should be, and Sophie adjusts the oxygen flow while asking him how his night was. He wheezes out a few words, clearly fatigued, and she encourages him to take deep breaths, though she knows it's more wishful thinking than practical advice.

Next, she sees Mrs. Whitmore, an ALS patient in her early 50s, who struggles with mobility and has just been fitted for a non-invasive ventilator. Sophie adjusts the straps carefully, making sure Mrs. Whitmore feels as comfortable as possible, knowing how quickly the disease can progress.

Mid-morning, she meets with Dr. Richards Malloy, a senior physician known for his clinical brilliance but sometimes quick decisions. As Sophie gives him a rundown of critical cases—oxygen levels, respiratory difficulties, responses to treatments—she finds herself internally questioning each diagnosis. Should they have increased Mr. Diaz's bronchodilator dosage sooner? Is Mrs. Whitmore's ventilator adjustment enough to prevent further decline?

"Whitmore's struggling with that ventilator, isn't she?" Dr. Richards asks, glancing at the chart.

"Yes," Sophie says, maintaining a professional tone. "I was thinking about trying a higher pressure setting, but I wanted to get your opinion first."

Richards nods, then makes a few notes, moving on quickly to the next case. But Sophie can't shake her internal doubts. She knows the treatments by heart, the guidelines, the protocols—but that doesn't stop her from questioning if they could be doing more, or if they're already too late.

She continues her rounds, double-checking equipment, adjusting medications, and silently replaying each patient's history in her mind. She catches herself hesitating before leaving Mr. Diaz's room, wondering if today will be the day his condition worsens drastically. It's these quiet moments, the pauses between tasks, where her internal struggle peaks. She questions every decision, every diagnosis—haunted by memories of Emily and the feeling that she missed something critical with her best friend.

Sophie finishes her shift with a sigh of relief but can't fully shake the weight of the day. But at the end of each exhausting day, when Sophie returns to her quiet apartment, the framed protest sign from Emily hangs prominently on her wall. She stares at it, reminding herself of the friend she lost and the fight she's still in, though she keeps those memories locked away, even from herself. As she heads home, she's already thinking about the research papers she wants to read, hoping for something new, something that could make a difference for the patients she sees every day. But deep down, she knows that each day will bring similar questions, similar struggles, and the haunting reminder that, despite her best efforts, some battles are harder to win than others.

...

Sophie walks into Ms. Dawson's room, her heart sinking the moment she sees her patient. Ms. Dawson, frail and gasping for breath, is in the final stages of COPD. Her face is pale, her skin thin, and her eyes sunken from exhaustion. The harsh rasp of her laboured breathing fills the small room, drowning out any other sound. Sophie can feel the weight of the oxygen tank that Ms. Dawson relies on, knowing it's the only thing keeping her alive for now. Ms. Dawson reminds Sophie too much of Emily—Emily, who had once been so full of life, who had collapsed during a protest with a similar struggle for breath. The memory hits Sophie like a punch every darn time, and guilt wells up in her chest. She feels it every time she sees Ms. Dawson. The helplessness of those final days with Emily floods back—Emily pushing herself too hard, coughing until she couldn't anymore, and Sophie, standing by, unable to save her best friend. Ms. Dawson tries to speak, but only a weak rasp escapes her lips. Sophie leans in closer, adjusting the nasal cannula that's supposed to help her breathe easier, though it feels like a small comfort in the face of an inevitable decline. "It's okay," Sophie whispers, though she knows it's not. She forces herself to smile, hiding the fear and frustration gnawing at her insides.

"Am I...gonna be okay?" Ms. Dawson asks between breaths, her voice barely audible. Her words mirror Emily's last question to Sophie, moments before she passed.

Sophie's throat tightens. She wants to tell Ms. Dawson the truth, that there's nothing left to be done, that the disease has stolen too much. But she can't. She doesn't have the strength to face her own helplessness, let alone Ms. Dawson's. "We're doing everything we can," Sophie says instead, her voice soft but hollow. The words feel empty, just as they did with Emily.

The guilt grows heavier with each visit. Ms. Dawson's condition deteriorates rapidly, and Sophie feels herself slipping into a familiar cycle of helplessness. She pushes herself harder, researching new treatment options late into the night, asking Dr. Richards for second opinions, looking for anything that might make a difference. But deep down, she knows the outcome won't change. It never does.

During a routine check of Ms. Dawson's vitals, Sophie watches as her patient's chest rises and falls unevenly. She adjusts the oxygen levels, but it feels like a futile gesture—just like it had with Emily. She clenches her jaw, trying to hold back tears. She wanted to save Emily, to do more, to find a way. And now, she wants to save Ms. Dawson, but the guilt that she couldn't do it for Emily haunts her.

After her shift, Sophie finds herself sitting in the break room, staring at her hands. The frustration builds inside her—why hadn't she found a way to help Emily? Could she have pushed harder for better treatments? Should she have caught the signs earlier? And now, with Ms. Dawson, she feels like she's watching history repeat itself, powerless once again. In a quiet moment, Ms. Dawson reaches out and grabs Sophie's hand. "Thank you," she whispers, her voice cracking under the weight of her condition. Sophie blinks back tears, squeezing her hand gently. "You're welcome," she says softly, but in her mind, all she can think is, *I'm sorry.*

...

At The Tipsy Oak, the dim lights cast long shadows, and the constant hum of conversation fills the room. Behind the bar, Amelia wipes down glasses with quick, precise motions, her sharp eyes landing on Jack slouched over in his usual spot. She raises an eyebrow as she approaches him, her mouth already forming the sarcastic remark she's been holding back for weeks.

"Look who's back," she says, her tone dripping with mock enthusiasm. "The guy who's got it all figured out. How's that five-year plan going, Jack?"

Jack glances up from his drink, his lips curling into a dry smirk. "Oh, it's going great. I've downgraded to a five-minute plan. Just trying to make it through the next round." He taps the rim of his glass, signalling for another drink.

Amelia rolls her eyes, pouring him a whiskey. "Sure, because drowning yourself in cheap liquor is definitely the way to fix all your problems. What's next, therapy with tequila?"

He chuckles under his breath, the sound low and tired. "Might give that a try. Seems like it's working for now."

She leans against the bar, arms crossed, not letting him off the hook. "You know, some people actually deal with their issues. They don't just sit at a bar and drink them away."

Jack raises his glass in a mock toast. "Here's to those people. May they continue to be overachievers."

Amelia lets out a snort, shaking her head. "You're a real piece of work, Matthews. What's next? Moving into that couch permanently? I'm sure Zach loves having you as his new pet."

Jack shrugs, not denying it. "Rent's cheap."

"Yeah, I bet. I'm surprised you haven't started paying him in IOUs written on napkins."

Jack grins, but the expression doesn't reach his eyes. "It's a work in progress. Haven't quite gotten that desperate."

Amelia pauses, her tone softening just a fraction. "You know, Jack, one of these days you might want to actually try living your life instead of coasting through it." He takes a sip of his drink, feeling the burn of the whiskey slide down his throat. "Maybe. But for now..." He gestures around the bar, offering her a half-smile. "This is about as good as it gets."

Amelia throws the rag over her shoulder and gives him a long, assessing look. "You're hopeless, you know that?" Jack laughs, the sound rough but genuine this time. "Yeah, I've been told." She walks away, muttering under her breath, but there's a flicker of a smile on her face. Amidst the chaos of his crumbling life, Jack clings to these moments—tiny, sarcastic exchanges that keep him grounded, even if they're just distractions.

As the nights at The Tipsy Oak stretch longer, Jack and Amelia's late-night chats begin to take on a rhythm of their own. The bar clears out, leaving only the lingering scent of spilled beer and the low hum of the jukebox. Amelia locks up while Jack stays behind, nursing what's left of his drink. The silence between them feels familiar now—comfortable, almost—but there's always a tension that hovers beneath the surface, unspoken.

Amelia finishes wiping down the counter, tossing her rag aside with a tired sigh. "So, what's it gonna be tonight, Jack? Deep thoughts or bad jokes?"

He glances at her from his stool, a lazy smirk playing on his lips. "Why not both? You know I'm full of surprises."

"Yeah, sure," she says, her eyes rolling but a smile tugging at the corners of her mouth. "Surprises like showing up late to your own life."

Jack chuckles softly, swirling his drink. "What can I say? Punctuality was never my strong suit."

Amelia leans against the bar, her gaze lingering on him longer than usual. "You ever gonna let me in on what's really going on with you, or are we just gonna keep pretending your life is one big joke?"

He tenses slightly but masks it with a shrug. "Not much to tell. Just your typical guy in a downward spiral, trying to figure out how to stop spinning."

She raises an eyebrow. "Typical, huh? You think every guy in this bar has the same sad backstory as you? They dropped out of PhD programs? They graduated in economics?"

Jack huffs a laugh, but there's no humour behind it. "Maybe not. But I bet they've all got their own versions of it."

Amelia watches him, her expression softening. "You know, I don't really care about all the tragic details, Jack. But it'd be nice if you stopped hiding behind all the sarcasm."

There's a beat of silence before Jack responds. "I'm not hiding. I'm just... keeping things simple."

"Simple," she repeats, her voice laced with disbelief. "Right. Because staying emotionally detached is the definition of simple."

He offers a small, half-hearted smile. "It works for me." Amelia sighs, crossing her arms over her chest. "You're impossible, you know that?"

Jack tilts his head, a playful glint in his eye. "Yeah, I've been told." But beneath the banter, there's a crack in Jack's usual defenses. He watches Amelia as she finishes cleaning up, her presence somehow making the bar feel less empty. There's something about these late-night moments—the way she challenges him without pushing too hard, the way her sharp tongue softens when she thinks he's not looking—that keeps him coming back. It's as if she sees through his armour, but doesn't try to rip it off. Instead, she stands at the edge, waiting for him to open up on his own terms.

As the months pass, their conversations grow longer, more personal. Amelia talks about her dreams of opening her own bar someday, her struggles with balancing work and life, and the customers who drive her crazy. Jack listens, offers his dry humour in return, but keeps the details of his past—Liam, Emily, Evan, Sophie, the pain—close to his chest. Still, there's a shift between them. A slow, subtle unraveling of the walls Jack's built around himself. Late one night, after they've both had a few too many drinks, Amelia leans in closer than usual.

"You know," she says quietly, her voice carrying an edge of vulnerability, "you don't have to go through whatever this is alone."

Jack meets her gaze, something stirring deep inside him that he's not ready to acknowledge. "I know." And for the first time in a long time, he starts to wonder if maybe, just maybe, letting someone in wouldn't be so bad after all.

Chapter 2: Helplessness

Sophie sits stiffly in a circle of mismatched chairs, her arms crossed tightly over her chest as if to shield herself from the raw emotions hanging in the air. The room is quiet except for the occasional sound of a tissue being pulled from a box, the soft murmur of voices blending together like white noise in the background. It's her first grief therapy session, and she feels out of place, like she's trespassing on something deeply private, even though she's here for the same reason as everyone else.

Across from her, Dr. Elena Parker, a calm, composed woman with gentle eyes, leads the group. She looks at Sophie with a kind of understanding that makes her skin crawl. Sophie shifts uncomfortably, avoiding eye contact.

"Sophie, you don't have to say anything if you're not ready," Dr. Parker says, her voice soft but firm. "Just being here is a step."

Sophie clenches her jaw, resisting the urge to walk out. She didn't want to be here. The idea of sitting in a room full of strangers, spilling her pain, seemed unbearable. But she had promised Dr. Richard she'd at least try. "Grief isn't something you can fix," Dr. Parker had told her during their first session together, a one-on-one meeting that left Sophie even more uncomfortable than she's now. "It's something you have to live with." But Sophie doesn't want to live with it. She wants it to go away, to stop clawing at her heart every time she thinks of Emily or Liam or anyone with not enough time left to live. She doesn't want to hear platitudes about time healing all wounds or the idea that everything happens for a reason. There's no reason good enough to explain losing the people she cares about most.

As the session drags on, Sophie listens to the others speak —an older man who lost his wife of 40 years, a young mother grieving her child, and a woman in her thirties talking about her sister's sudden death. The words blur together, stories of heartbreak and loss weaving a fabric of shared pain. Yet Sophie still feels like an outsider.

When it's her turn to speak, Dr. Parker turns to her with a gentle nod. "Would you like to share, Sophie?"

Sophie's throat tightens, her pulse quickening. She shakes her head quickly. "No. Not today."

Dr. Parker doesn't push, simply offering a small, understanding smile. "That's okay. There's no rush. Grief is on its own timeline."

Sophie forces a tight smile, but inside, she feels a storm brewing. What timeline? She doesn't want to wait. The grief, the guilt, the present, the memories—they're suffocating her, and talking about it feels like pouring salt in an open wound. She feels the weight of the loss pressing down on her chest like a heavy stone she can't move.

After the session ends, Sophie is the first to leave, bolting out the door into the cold air. She takes a deep breath, her hands trembling as she reaches for her phone. She almost calls Jack, the one who'll understand, but stops herself. He's dealing with his own grief, and the last thing he needs is her dragging him further into the darkness. Instead, she walks back to her apartment in silence, her thoughts racing. Maybe Dr. Parker was right—grief isn't something you can fix. But Sophie can't help feeling like she's broken, stuck in a cycle of pain that has no end.

At work, Sophie walks through the bustling hallways of St. Luke's Medical Center, her gaze fixed ahead, expertly avoiding the usual chatter between nurses and doctors. She doesn't stop by the nurse's station to catch up or share a coffee, nor does she engage in the small moments of camaraderie that typically fill the day. Her colleagues have grown used to her silence, but some still shoot her concerned looks as she passes by.

She heads straight to the break room during her lunch hour, but instead of eating or relaxing, she pulls out her tablet, opening up the soft copy Emily's old medical records. Her lunch sits untouched as she scans through each line of treatment, flipping back and forth between diagnostic notes, test results, and prescriptions. The weight of every moment hits her like a punch to the gut—the hospital visits, the oxygen therapy, Emily's persistent cough, the signs that maybe, just maybe, Sophie should have caught sooner. She feels a constant need to check and recheck, as if somewhere within the pages, there's an answer she overlooked—a clue that might explain why they couldn't stop Emily's rapid decline. Dr. Richards, now her supervising physician, sticks his head into the break room at one point, noticing Sophie's usual focused expression. "You ever take a break, Sophie?" he asks with a half-smile.

Sophie forces a smile in return, one that doesn't reach her eyes. "Just catching up on some research," she responds, keeping her voice neutral.

Dr. Richards shakes his head, half-amused, half-worried. "Well, don't bury yourself in it. You can't change the past."

Sophie nods absently, but as soon as he's gone, her attention returns to Emily's records. She finds herself fixating on the smallest details—Emily's breathing patterns, the decline in her lung function, the medications prescribed. She scrolls to the last visit, where the words "end-stage COPD" are typed in clinical detachment, and her stomach twists. She clicks through to the prescription notes: long-term oxygen therapy, bronchodilators, inhaled corticosteroids, all the medications that had once given them a glimmer of hope. Sophie remembers the long days spent together, Emily joking between gasps for air, trying to lighten the heaviness in the room. And now, all that remains are these cold, sterile documents that offer no comfort, only reminders of what was lost. The guilt creeps in, sharper with every read-through. Did she miss something vital? Could they have pushed for more aggressive treatment sooner? Every time Sophie reexamines the records, she's searching for some explanation, but all she finds are more questions. She knows it's irrational—but the doubt won't leave her. Her lunch break ends, and she closes Emily's file with a resigned sigh. She stands up, pulling her hair into a tight ponytail, and heads back into the ward to finish her shift, carrying the weight of her grief like a shadow that never leaves her side.

Sophie sits at her desk late into the evening, staring at Emily's prescription notes for what feels like the hundredth time. The fluorescent light above flickers slightly, casting a dull glow over the room. As she scrolls through the medication history, her eyes land on a note she had somehow skimmed over before—or maybe she just didn't want to acknowledge it. Emily had been prescribed inhalers—bronchodilators to open up her airways, corticosteroids to reduce inflammation—but the notes indicated that she hadn't been using them regularly in the last few months before her death. Sophie's heart clenches as she reads the reminder in the records: "Patient reports inconsistent use of prescribed inhalers." She closes her eyes, feeling a wave of nausea. How did she miss this? She was with Emily every day, yet her friend never mentioned skipping doses. Maybe she was trying to keep her spirits up, hiding how much she was struggling with the daily regimen. Emily had always been stubborn, especially during the protests, pushing herself far beyond her limits. And Sophie had let it happen, standing by her side, thinking Emily's strength would carry her through. But now, reading that Emily hadn't been adhering to her inhalers, Sophie feels an overwhelming sense of failure. She had been right there, helping Emily fight, yet she missed this crucial detail that might have prolonged her life—or at least made her more comfortable in her final months. The knowledge of it claws at her, feeding her guilt and regret. Sophie can hear Emily's voice in her mind, joking about how annoying it was to keep track of the inhalers. Emily had hated being dependent on medication, hated the constant reminders that her body was failing her. But Sophie should have known better. She should have insisted, pushed harder, reminded Emily every day if she had to. She feels like she failed her friend when it mattered most. Her eyes blur with unshed tears as she replays those final months in her mind, wondering if she could have done something—anything—to make things different. Could she have noticed and confronted Emily sooner? Would it have made a difference if Emily had used her inhalers more consistently? Sophie slams the tablet closed and buries her head in her hands, the weight of guilt suffocating her. The report is over five hundred pages long, then there's her own research and she's sick of it but her mind won't listen. She thought she had come to terms with Emily's death, but this—this small but significant oversight—feels like a betrayal. One she can't forgive herself for.

...

Jack sits in a corner booth at *The Green Bean*, the cafe outside the college, where they used to meet before everything fell apart. His fingers trace the edges of the worn group photo he keeps in his wallet—a photo of him, Sophie, Liam, Evan, Madison and Emily during better times, laughing outside the café with their arms around each other. The image is faded, but the memories feel even more distant, like a different lifetime. His eyes linger on Liam's carefree grin, the kind that once seemed unshakable, and Emily's bright, determined gaze that always hinted at something fierce.

Jack feels nothing but an empty hollowness as he sips his now-cold coffee, drowning in the silence that surrounds him despite the bustling café. He's been here for hours, pretending to read the book he brought, but in reality, he's stuck in his own head, resisting the idea that he should move forward—that healing is even an option. Suddenly, a loud voice cuts through his trance.

"Jack! Man, is that you?"

Jack looks up and sees Mason, one of Liam's and his college friend, standing by his table with a wide grin. Mason's hair is a mess, his clothes are slightly mismatched, and he's holding a cup of coffee that sloshes dangerously close to spilling. The sight of him is both jarring and oddly comforting. Mason, with his strange, chaotic energy, had always been an oddball, the one who cracked the weirdest jokes in the middle of serious conversations.

"Yeah, it's me," Jack mutters, trying to force a smile that doesn't quite reach his eyes.

Mason slides into the seat across from him without hesitation, completely ignoring the fact that Jack clearly wasn't in the mood for company. "Wow, haven't seen you in ages. This place brings back memories, huh? Good times. Well, except for the terrible coffee—seriously, why do we keep coming back here?" Jack lets out a dry chuckle, surprised at himself. Mason always had a way of getting under your skin with his quirky humour, but somehow, it worked. "Still the same awful jokes, I see," Jack says, shaking his head.

"What can I say? I'm consistent," Mason replies with a grin, leaning back in his chair. "But hey, seriously—how've you been? Haven't seen you since... well, since..."

Jack knows what Mason is about to say but doesn't need to hear it. He cuts him off, the numbness creeping back into his voice. "Yeah, it's been a while."

Mason looks at him for a moment, his usual lightheartedness faltering. "You look... different. Everything okay?" Jack shrugs, not knowing how to respond. He's tired of people asking him that question, tired of pretending like he's fine. But Mason's oddball energy somehow makes it easier to deflect. "I'm still here. That's something, right?" Mason leans forward, elbows on the table, his expression softening. "Look, I get it. It's been rough for all of us. But you can't keep… I don't know… just going through the motions like this."

Jack stiffens, hating the direction of the conversation. He's been doing everything he can to avoid thinking too deeply about what's next, about how he's supposed to "heal" or "move on." The idea feels impossible, like an insult to everything he went through and is still going.

"I don't need a pep talk, Mason," Jack says, his voice edged with irritation.

Mason holds up his hands in mock surrender. "Whoa, no pep talk here, dude. Just… saying I'm here. And, you know, maybe a bad joke or two to jolt you back to life."

Jack sighs, but a part of him—however small—appreciates the effort. He glances down at the photo again, a weight pressing on his chest. He wants to let go, to stop carrying the guilt and the memories like anchors, but something inside him resists. Healing feels like betrayal.

Mason notices the photo in Jack's hand and taps the table. "Hey, remember that time Liam convinced Emily that the café's secret ingredient in the cookies was cayenne pepper?"

Jack chuckles, this time genuinely. "Yeah, and she actually believed him until she took a bite and realized they were just regular chocolate chip."

Mason laughs, the sound loud and carefree. "Man, Liam could sell anything with that charm of his. It's hard not to miss that guy."

Jack nods, but the heaviness in his chest doesn't lift. He misses Liam, more than he can put into words, but talking about it—about past and himself now—just makes the void feel bigger.

Mason's laughter fades, and for a moment, they sit in silence, the weight of everything unsaid settling between them. Jack knows Mason's trying to help, in his own weird way, but Jack isn't ready to heal yet. He isn't sure he ever will be. "Thanks for the company, Mason," Jack finally says, standing up and stuffing the photo back into his wallet. "But I've gotta go."

Mason looks like he wants to say more, but he just nods, his usual grin slipping. "Take care, Jack. And, hey, if you ever want to grab a terrible cup of coffee again, you know where to find me." Jack gives a half-hearted wave, feeling just as disconnected as before. Mason's jokes may have shaken him for a moment, but the numbness quickly returns. The path to healing and getting out of depression, if there even is one, still feels miles away. As Jack stands to leave the café, Mason casually brings up Liam's unrelenting passion for life. "You know, Liam never gave up on anything. Even when things got tough, he just… fought. Like he always had this fire in him." Those words hit Jack like a freight train, freezing him in place. His jaw tightens, his fists clench, and a wave of guilt rushes over him, nearly suffocating. Liam's fire, Liam's fight —it all sounds so distant, so unreachable now, like a cruel reminder of Jack's own failure to keep that fire alive for himself.

"You have no idea what you're talking about," Jack mutters, his voice low, dangerous.

Mason looks taken aback, not expecting the sudden shift in Jack's demeanour. "Hey, man, I didn't mean anything by it. I'm just saying—Liam wouldn't want you to—"

"Shut up, Mason!" Jack explodes, his voice louder than he intended, causing a few heads to turn in the café. His heart pounds in his chest, his vision narrowing as his anger spirals out of control. "You think I don't know that? You think I don't *know* what Liam would've wanted? Stop acting like you understand. You weren't there."

Mason's face pales, his hands raised in surrender. "Jack, I didn't mean to—" But Jack's too far gone, the guilt that's been gnawing at him for months finally boiling over. He can feel the walls closing in, the suffocating weight of it all pressing down on him. He should've been the economics professor or something. He should've done more. He wasn't enough. He wasn't strong enough. And now he was almost dead, and it was all his fault.

The thoughts race through his mind faster than he can control them, his breathing quickening, turning ragged. He pushes past Mason, nearly knocking over his coffee, and stumbles out of the café, the cold air outside doing nothing to quell the rising panic inside him. His chest tightens, his hands trembling as he grips the edge of a nearby bench. His breaths come in shallow gasps, each one more laboured than the last. Jack feels like he's drowning, like there's no air left in the world, and the guilt is dragging him under.

He presses his palms against his head, trying to steady himself, but the panic only deepens. His vision blurs, and all he can hear is the echo of Mason's voice and the terrible, undeniable truth—he failed. He failed. He failed himself and everyone around him. And now he's alone, stuck in the aftermath of it all, unable to fix it, unable to keep moving.

A few pedestrians glance at him as they pass by, but Jack is too lost in the panic to notice. He crouches down by the bench, knees to his chest, desperately trying to catch his breath, his mind spinning out of control. He can't breathe. He can't think. All he can feel is the crushing weight of guilt and loss suffocating him. Minutes pass, though they feel like hours, and eventually, his breathing slows, his heart still pounding but no longer threatening to burst out of his chest. Jack pulls himself up slowly, his body shaking as he leans against the bench, the panic receding but leaving behind a hollow, aching emptiness. He doesn't go back into the café. He can't face Mason, or anyone, right now. Instead, Jack drags himself down the street, his feet heavy, his head pounding with the aftershocks of his panic attack. He walks aimlessly, unsure of where he's going, but knowing that wherever it is, it's far away from the weight of his guilt, if only for a moment.

Chapter 3: Breakdowns

Jack's life begins to spiral even further as the panic attacks become more frequent and intense. The tightness in his chest, the overwhelming sense of dread, and the racing thoughts consume him more often than not. He feels trapped inside his own mind, unable to breathe or think clearly. His daily routine becomes one of avoidance—of emotions, of memories, of people. Jack spends more time at *The Tipsy Oak*, throwing back shots of whiskey, trying to drown the anxiety that gnaws at him. He's feeling weakest he felt in his life.

He avoids talking about what he's going through. His friends notice the change in him, the growing distance. Zach, his old childhood friend who lets Jack crash on his couch, tries to get him to open up, but every attempt is met with a shrug or a deflecting joke. Jack's humour, once sharp and dry, now serves as a mask to cover the cracks in his façade. The more he drinks, the more isolated he feels, even when surrounded by people.

On particularly bad night after a panic attack leaves him breathless and curled up on the floor, Jack begrudgingly makes a doctor's appointment. He sits in the sterile office, barely listening as the doctor goes over his symptoms. Jack's leg bounces restlessly, his mind wandering as the doctor mentions "anxiety disorder" and "panic attacks."

"I'm going to prescribe you something for the anxiety," the doctor says, scribbling on a pad. "It'll help you manage the symptoms, but you'll need to follow up regularly and consider therapy as well."

Jack glances at the prescription slip—anti-anxiety medication, something to help with the panic attacks. He nods absently, stuffing the paper into his pocket without a second thought. But deep down, he already knows he won't fill it. Taking the meds feels like admitting defeat, like acknowledging the fact that he's losing control. And Jack can't bring himself to face that. Instead, he continues to self-medicate with alcohol, pretending the panic isn't there, even as it threatens to swallow him whole. His insomnia worsens, the nights stretching longer as he lies awake, staring at the ceiling, his mind racing with thoughts of the life he feels slipping away from himself.

He doesn't go to his uncle Dr. Richards on purpose, he don't want to get inspired or be a topic of degradation amongst family and relatives. During his visit with Dr. Nguyen, a soft-spoken but firm general practitioner, Jack barely listens as the doctor goes over the risks of self-medicating with alcohol. Dr. Nguyen knows Jack's type—someone who refuses to acknowledge the depth of their pain, relying on destructive habits to cope.

"Jack, I'm seeing some red flags here," Dr. Nguyen begins, reviewing Jack's recent health complaints. "Your migraines, insomnia, and these panic attacks—they're serious. Alcohol might numb you for a bit, but it's only making things worse. It can cause rebound anxiety, increase your risk of depression, and worsen your sleep issues."

Jack shifts uncomfortably in his chair, running a hand through his disheveled hair. He's not in the mood for a lecture, especially ones he's heard before.

"Yeah, yeah," he mutters, shrugging off the warning, his eyes darting toward the window. "I've got it under control. Just a drink here and there to take the edge off."

Dr. Nguyen presses on, unwilling to let Jack's nonchalant attitude go unchecked. "You may think it's helping, but alcohol's a depressant. Combine that with your anxiety, and you're putting your health—and your life—at risk. Your body's already strained from the insomnia and migraines. And if you keep avoiding treatment, you're heading down a dangerous road."

Dr. Nguyen pulls out the same prescription pad from earlier, jotting down another reminder for Jack's anti-anxiety medication. "This is something to help you manage your panic attacks and anxiety. But it only works if you take it, Jack. I can't force you, but you need to take this seriously. And therapy would help too."

Jack takes the new slip of paper, shoving it into his jacket pocket where it joins the first prescription he's been ignoring for weeks. The paper crumples into the fabric, out of sight and out of mind. As Jack leaves the doctor's office, he knows deep down that Dr. Nguyen is right. But the thought of actually addressing his emotions, taking the meds, or going to therapy —it all feels like too much. So instead, he heads back to *The Tipsy Oak* for another drink, numbing himself for just a little longer, the prescription remaining buried in his pocket, untouched.

...

Sophie's emotional breakdown comes like a wave she didn't see coming. Oliver, a young boy newly admitted to her ward with ALS, reminds her of everything she's been trying to suppress. He's just eight years old but already has that same brave, stubborn fight that Liam had. The boy smiles through his pain, always quick with a joke despite the challenges he faces. But for Sophie, every interaction with him feels like a stab to the heart. One evening, after an exhausting shift, Sophie finds herself in Oliver's room, helping him adjust his breathing equipment. His soft voice cuts through the beeps of the machines, and he asks, "Do you think I'll get to play soccer again someday?"

Sophie freezes. For a second, she's transported back to Liam, lying in his hospital bed, making dark jokes about his wheelchair and asking questions that neither of them could answer. It's too familiar, too raw. She holds back tears as she helps Oliver settle in, telling him softly, "I hope so, Oliver. I really do." But the hope in her words feels hollow. Later, after she's finished her rounds, she finds herself in the hospital's staff breakroom, her mind spinning. The weight of her unresolved grief presses down on her like a vice. She thinks about Emily, about Liam, about over hundred patients diagnosed with fatal diseases—about how she wasn't able to save any of them despite everything she did. And now, here she is again, watching another young life slowly being taken by the same cruel disease.

The dam finally breaks. Sophie barely makes it to the bathroom before collapsing into sobs. She leans against the cold tiles, her hands shaking as she covers her face, struggling to catch her breath. The guilt she's been carrying for so long overwhelms her. She couldn't save Emily, couldn't save Liam. And now, looking at Oliver, she feels that same helplessness all over again. As the tears flow, she whispers to herself, "I should've done more. I should've been better at my research." But deep down, Sophie knows there was nothing more she could've done. ALS and COPD are relentless diseases. Still, the guilt clings to her like a second skin, and she wonders if she'll ever be able to let it go. She returns back to the duty.

Sophie's hands tremble slightly as she adjusts Oliver's breathing mask. The hiss of the oxygen machine fills the room, echoing memories of the same sound that accompanied Emily's final weeks. She watches the numbers on the monitor closely—oxygen saturation levels, heart rate—everything needs to be stable. Her mind flashes back to those nights of countless worries by Emily's side, when every dip in oxygen sent a surge of panic through her veins. Oliver looks up at her, wide-eyed but trusting, as she carefully administers his breathing treatment. His little chest rises and falls steadily, but each puff of air that escapes through the mask tugs at Sophie's heartstrings. She reminds herself to focus—this isn't Emily. She can't afford to slip into the past now, not when Oliver needs her to stay present. Still, every beep of the monitor seems louder than it should be, every number on the screen drags her back to those final, desperate days with Emily. She can almost hear Emily's laboured breaths, see the pale, exhausted face staring up at her as Sophie helplessly tried to manage her symptoms. With each update to Oliver's treatment plan—changing the dosage of his medications, adjusting the flow of his oxygen, carefully logging his progress—Sophie feels the weight of her grief pressing harder on her chest. She's following the same protocols, charting the same patterns, reliving every agonizing step of the decline. The reminders are unavoidable. After leaving Oliver's room, Sophie rushes to the nearest empty hallway, her breath shallow. Her mind screams that she's somehow failing again.

...

At The Tipsy Oak, the usual late-night crowd had thinned out, leaving Jack and Amelia to close up. Jack was wiping down the bar, his mind lost in its usual fog of memories. Amelia, leaning against the counter, eyed him with her typical sharp look.

"You gonna talk about your dead friend tonight, or are you cleaning the puke bucket?" she asked, half-smiling as she threw the challenge his way.

Jack shot her a glance, unamused. "I'll take the puke bucket," he muttered, grabbing the mop with a reluctant sigh.

Amelia chuckled, leaning back, clearly enjoying the discomfort she caused. "You always take the puke bucket. One of these days, you're gonna run out of excuses, Jack."

He shook his head, dragging the mop across the sticky floor. "One of these days," he echoed, though they both knew he wasn't ready for that day yet. For now, the puke bucket was easier than facing the ghosts waiting in the corners of his mind.

As he bent down, cleaning with exaggerated effort, he smirked, throwing back, "You know, you could help, considering this was probably your doing."

Amelia raised her hands in mock defence. "Hey, you're the one avoiding the heart-to-heart. Not my fault puke is your emotional safe space." Despite himself, Jack let out a quiet laugh. For a moment, the weight of everything lightened, if only just a bit.

Chapter 4: Big Pain, Small Steps

After running into Mason again at The Green Bean, Jack found himself returning to the café more often, despite the memories it stirred. The place still held echoes of Liam, Evan and Emily, but it also became a small refuge, a space to avoid the darkness that filled his apartment and the bar's suffocating atmosphere. Mason joined him upon the invitation, as usual, with his quirky jokes and irreverent energy. Over coffee, Mason casually mentioned his involvement in a volunteer program at the local community centre, where he helped run grief workshops for teens.

"You should come by, man. We could use someone with your...experience," Mason said, a mix of genuine concern and awkwardness in his voice.

Jack scoffed, stirring his coffee. "Yeah, I'm not exactly in a position to give anyone advice on grief or depression." Mason shrugged, leaning back in his chair. "You'd be surprised. Sometimes just showing up is enough. Besides, it's not like they need Dr. Phil. Just someone who gets it."

At first, Jack waved off the idea. The last thing he wanted was to confront his own feelings and emotions by helping someone else with theirs. But after another long night of drinking and self-loathing at The Tipsy Oak, he found himself texting Mason the next morning: *I'll stop by the centre. No promises.*

When he arrived at the community centre, Jack felt out of place, unsure what he had to offer. The room was small, filled with mostly teenagers who looked like they'd rather be anywhere else. But something about their distant expressions reminded him of himself—the numbness, the silent weight they carried.

As the first session went on, Jack didn't say much, just observed as Mason led the discussion. It wasn't until one of the teens, a quiet girl named Jenna, shared a story about losing her brother that Jack finally spoke up. The words came slowly at first, but as he talked about past, about the guilt and the jokes and the silences that never got filled, he realized how much he had buried inside. He advised them to not let the life pass them by as it has happened with himself. After the workshop, Mason patted Jack on the back. "See? Told you. Just showing up." Jack wasn't sure he was ready to fully confront his grief, but the act of helping others, even in small ways, gave him a sense of purpose he hadn't felt in a long time. It was something—maybe not everything—but enough to keep him coming back. As Jack continued attending the coping workshops, he quickly realized that teenagers had a brutal honesty he wasn't prepared for. On one particularly awkward afternoon, one of the teens, a lanky boy named Trevor, blurted out, "So, you're like…the sad bartender guy, right? You were bright student once but you failed in practical life after that?"

The room fell silent for a moment, and Jack felt his face flush. "Uh, I guess so," he mumbled, scratching the back of his neck.

"Dude, that's kind of your thing now," another teen, Sara, chimed in with a smirk. "Like, the guy who pours drinks and gives sad life advice."

Jack chuckled, shaking his head. "Well, if you need drink recipes, I'm your guy. Life advice? Probably not your best bet."

The group laughed, and the tension that always lingered in those sessions eased up. Jack's awkwardness, his fumbling attempts to connect, somehow made the room lighter. Over time, the teens embraced it, often turning his self-deprecating humour into a way to break the ice.

"You're not just the sad bartender guy," Mason said after one session. "You're like… the sad bartender guy with a heart of gold."

Jack rolled his eyes but smiled. "Yeah, well, don't expect too much gold. I'm more like a rusty bottle opener at this point." But it worked. His awkward, self-aware humour became a part of the healing process for the group. They laughed at his mishaps, and in return, Jack found a small bit of healing himself—through sarcasm, shared stories, and the unexpected connection that came with being "the sad bartender guy."

...

Sophie's project began quietly, almost as a personal endeavour to cope with her indecision, but it soon turned into something bigger. She started by designing simple pamphlets about ALS—detailing symptoms, treatments, and the importance of early diagnosis. Each page was filled with facts that she wished more people had known during Emily's battle. While sitting in the hospital's break room one evening, she nervously approached Nate, a fellow nurse known for his practical yet warm demeanour. He was flipping through patient charts when Sophie slid a rough draft of her pamphlet across the table.

"I'm working on this ALS awareness project," she explained, her voice steady but soft. "It's in memory of Emily and those we lost, but I want it to be something real, something that can make a difference."

Nate looked up, then down at the pamphlet, skimming through the pages. "This is good, Sophie," he said, nodding approvingly. "Really good. You know, I've been thinking we need more than just handouts. How about a walk? A fundraising event to get people involved?" The idea hit Sophie like a spark. A walk in memory of Emily. She could already envision it—hundreds of people walking through the city, raising awareness and funds for ALS research.

"You'd help?" she asked, surprised by his enthusiasm.

“Of course. This kind of thing is important,” Nate said, giving her a reassuring smile. “We could gather volunteers, reach out to local businesses, maybe even get a few sponsors. Plus, I know someone who’s great with organizing these things.”

For the first time in months, Sophie felt a glimmer of excitement—a new purpose that didn’t just revolve around grief. It was a way to keep Emily’s spirit alive, to turn her pain into something positive. She and Nate spent their breaks brainstorming, gathering resources, and planning the walk. Slowly but surely, the project took shape, and Sophie found herself more inspired.

Sophie and Nate’s partnership grew naturally, as they spent more time together planning the ALS awareness walk. Despite Sophie’s insistence on keeping things strictly professional, there was an undeniable connection forming between them—though she wasn’t ready to acknowledge it.

It started with little things. Nate’s gentle teasing became a constant thread in their interactions, lightening Sophie’s otherwise heavy days. One afternoon, as they were poring over potential routes for the walk, Nate leaned over the map and squinted dramatically.

“I think we should add a pit stop here,” he said, pointing to a café. “You know, just in case people need emergency coffee. Especially you. I’ve seen you after a night shift.” Sophie looked up, her lips twitching into a reluctant smile. “Oh, really? And what do I look like after a night shift?” “Like a zombie in scrubs. But you’re a very efficient zombie, I’ll give you that.”

Sophie chuckled, a sound that felt foreign yet comforting. It was the first real laugh she’d had in months, and Nate noticed it too. His teasing wasn't intrusive; it was always just enough to lift her spirits without making her uncomfortable. Over time, these moments of levity began to chip away at the emotional wall Sophie had built around herself. During their planning meetings, Nate would find subtle ways to make her smile. When Sophie suggested making the pamphlets more visually engaging, Nate mockingly offered to add cartoon lungs with superhero capes, calling it "COPD: The Reckoning." Sophie rolled her eyes but laughed, appreciating his effort to keep things light.

Despite Nate's warmth, Sophie was still emotionally raw, struggling to balance herself with the task at hand. She often caught herself zoning out during their meetings, lost in memories and thoughts. Nate, sensing when she needed space, never pushed. But he was always there—steady, patient, offering support without expectation. One evening, after a particularly long day at the hospital, Sophie and Nate were wrapping up their meeting in the break room. The conversation had turned personal, but Sophie instinctively steered it back to work.

"You know, we're making a lot of progress with this walk," she said, avoiding his gaze as she shuffled through her notes. "Emily would've... she would've loved this."

Nate leaned back in his chair, watching her closely. "You're doing something incredible, Sophie. But you don't always have to hide behind the project."

Sophie stiffened, her guard instantly going up. "I'm not hiding," she said quickly, her voice tighter than she intended. "I just want to make sure it's perfect."

Nate didn't push, but his eyes softened with understanding. "I know. Just... remember to take care of yourself, too." For a moment, they sat in silence, the unspoken tension hanging between them. Sophie knew Nate cared about her—not just as a colleague but as something more. And while she wasn't ready for anything beyond friendship, she couldn't deny how much his presence meant to her.

As weeks passed, their late-night planning sessions became routine. After one long evening, Nate handed her a cup of coffee with a smirk. "Zombie Sophie needs fuel." Sophie smiled, shaking her head. "You're insufferable, you know that?" "But I make good coffee," he replied with a grin, earning another small laugh from her. It was moments like these—quiet, simple, yet filled with warmth—that Sophie found herself drawn to. Even though she wasn't ready for romance, Nate's gentle humour and steadfast support were slowly helping her heal. His presence was a balm, soothing the ache she felt from losing Emily and Liam, even if she wasn't fully aware of it yet. Nate never crossed any lines. He respected her boundaries, understanding that Sophie was still navigating the storm of her emotions. But his care was evident in every interaction—the way he listened, the way he encouraged her, and the way he gave her space when she needed it. And for Sophie, that was more than enough.

Chapter 5: Facing the Lost

One late, cold night, Jack found himself sprawled across Zach's old, sagging couch, a half-empty bottle of whiskey on the table in front of him. The apartment was quiet except for the faint hum of the fridge and the occasional drip from the leaky faucet. His head pounded from too much alcohol, his thoughts swirling in a haze of guilt and regret. He fumbled for his phone, intending to drown his thoughts in mindless noise, but instead, he stumbled upon an old recording—Liam's band. His thumb hovered over the play button for a moment, hesitation gnawing at him, before he finally gave in and pressed it. The familiar sound of Liam's voice filled the room, raw and unpolished but full of passion. It was a live recording from a college show they had all attended—back when things were simpler, before illnesses had torn everything apart.

The opening chords hit Jack like a freight train, immediately sending him spiralling back into memories of Liam on stage, his fingers gliding effortlessly over the strings of his guitar. Jack had always admired Liam's talent, his ability to capture a room's attention with just a few notes. Now, hearing that voice again felt like a punch to the gut.

Jack closed his eyes, letting the music wash over him. At first, he tried to shut it out, to numb himself with another swig of whiskey. But the more he listened, the more the weight of it all bore down on him—the pain, the loss, the guilt. Memories flooded his mind—Liam's jokes in the hospital, the road trips they never took, the way Liam had faced his illness with a strength Jack couldn't fathom. Suddenly, the numbness he had been chasing for years cracked, and Jack broke down. Tears streamed down his face, silent at first, then full-bodied sobs that he couldn't control. He clutched the phone in his hand, the music still playing, Liam's voice echoing in his ears. Jack's chest tightened as the overwhelming sense of loss consumed him. He had been running from that and from himself for so long—running from the guilt of surviving, from the grief that threatened to swallow him whole.

"I should've been something, I had talent but I didn't use it. I became a damn addict. Now I'm depressed. He didn't had time to do the things he wished. I've it all and I didn't do it." Jack choked out to the empty room, his voice barely above a whisper. "I should've done more."

He had always felt like he had failed himself and everyone around him, like he hadn't fought hard enough, hadn't been the person he needed himself to be. Jack realized he wasn't just grieving Liam's death; he was mourning his own failures. He had spent so much time avoiding that guilt—drowning it in alcohol, pushing away those who cared—but now, there was no escaping it. The song played on, and Jack let it. He let himself feel the rawness of the grief, the guilt that he had buried deep inside. For the first time since Liam's death, he allowed himself to confront the pain instead of running from it. The realization hit him hard—he wasn't just angry at the world for taking Liam; he was angry at himself for not being enough, for not saving himself, for not knowing how to. Jack's sobs subsided into quiet tears as the song came to an end. The silence that followed felt heavy, but also strangely freeing. He knew he couldn't keep running. Liam's death wasn't something he could outrun or drink away. The only way out was through it. Wiping his face with the sleeve of his jacket, Jack sat up, staring blankly at the phone in his hand. He knew what he had to do—he had to stop running, stop numbing, and start facing the depression head-on.

...

After the emotional breakdown with Liam's music playing, Jack made a decision he had been avoiding for far too long. A few days later, he found himself in Dr. Nguyen's office, the sterile scent of antiseptic in the air. He sat stiffly in the chair across from her, staring at the diplomas on the wall, fidgeting with Liam's old guitar pick in his hand. His exhaustion was written all over his face—dark circles under his eyes, disheveled hair, and the weight of sleepless nights hung heavy on him. Dr. Nguyen sat quietly, her pen poised as she looked over Jack's chart. She had seen this all before—the over-reliance on alcohol, the neglect of prescribed treatments, the avoidance of therapy. Jack was yet another patient trying to run from pain.

"Jack," she said gently, "I see you haven't filled your prescription for the anti-anxiety meds." Jack shrugged, avoiding eye contact. "Didn't think they'd help much."

She studied him for a moment before speaking. "You've been through a lot. It's not uncommon to feel like the meds won't make a difference, but they're just one piece of the puzzle. You're dealing with insomnia, anxiety, and grief. This isn't something you should face alone or try to medicate with alcohol."

Jack shifted uncomfortably. He wasn't used to opening up about his emotions, especially with a doctor. Dr. Nguyen leaned forward, her tone firm but understanding. "If you keep self-medicating with alcohol, your body will pay the price, and it won't help in the long run. Let's talk about a plan."

Jack listened quietly as she explained her approach. She adjusted his medication, lowering the dosage of the sleeping pills to avoid dependency, but added a selective serotonin reuptake inhibitor (SSRI) to help manage his anxiety and depression more effectively. She stressed the importance of consistency and gradual improvement, reminding him that there wouldn't be any quick fixes.

"The real work," Dr. Nguyen continued, "is in therapy. I'm recommending grief counselling along with cognitive-behavioural therapy (CBT). You're not just dealing with insomnia and anxiety, Jack. You're carrying a lot of unresolved thoughts."

He winced but nodded. "I've been having nightmares," he admitted, his voice barely above a whisper. "About him... about how I couldn't help him."

Dr. Nguyen met his gaze, her expression empathetic. "It's common to have nightmares when you're processing traumatic loss. The therapy will help you work through those feelings, the guilt, and the grief."

Jack swallowed hard, knowing she was right. She handed him the revised prescription and the number of a therapist specializing in coping and grief therapy. He stared at the paper in his hands for a long moment before finally stuffing it into his pocket.

"Take it one day at a time, Jack. You don't have to carry this weight on your own," Dr. Nguyen said softly as he stood to leave.

That night, Jack sat in his small, cluttered apartment, staring at the untouched bottle of whiskey on the counter. Instead of reaching for it, he grabbed the prescription and texted the therapist. It was the first step—small, hesitant—but it was a step forward. When Jack began his therapy sessions, he approached them reluctantly. Sitting in the sterile office with Dr. Parker, his therapist, felt awkward at first. The walls were lined with books and plants, a sharp contrast to the cold hospital room he remembered Liam in. The first few sessions were filled with silence, Jack not quite ready to talk. But eventually, the nightmares forced his hand. He started talking about Liam—about the moments in the hospital, the road trip they never took, then he did it with Sophie, and the overwhelming guilt he feels for surviving this far. Dr. Parker listened intently, gently guiding him through the process of confronting those buried emotions. "You can't change what happened, Jack. But we can work on accepting it." The sessions were hard. Reliving the hospital scenes, Liam's final moments, and the jokes Liam made about his own condition was agonizing. But slowly, through therapy, Jack began to understand that his guilt, while deeply painful, wasn't something he had to shoulder alone. The medication and therapy began working together, helping him manage the insomnia, the anxiety, and—most of all—the depression he's in.

...

Sophie sat stiffly in her therapist Dr. Elena Parker's office, hands clenched in her lap, her eyes fixed on the small plant sitting on the windowsill. She had been coming to these sessions for weeks now, but each time felt like a battle. Dr. Parker was kind, patient, and always softly encouraging Sophie to let her guard down, but the words Sophie needed to say felt stuck in her throat. Today, though, something was different. The memory had been bubbling at the surface for days, clawing to be spoken. Dr. Parker's voice was gentle. "You've been thinking about Emily a lot recently. What's been on your mind?"

Sophie bit her lip, feeling the knot in her chest tighten. "I can't stop thinking about her last few days," she said, her voice barely above a whisper. Dr. Parker nodded, allowing her to continue at her own pace.

"I was there," Sophie began, her hands twisting the fabric of her scrubs as she spoke. "I was her nurse, her friend, and I thought… I thought I could save her, somehow. But I couldn't."

She paused, the memory of the hospital flooding back. "Her blood oxygen levels kept dropping, no matter what we did. She was on oxygen, then the ventilator, but it wasn't enough. I watched her struggle to breathe, and I felt so... helpless." Sophie's breath hitched, and her eyes brimmed with unshed tears. "I'm a nurse. I'm supposed to help people get better. But I couldn't help her. I couldn't fix it."

Dr. Parker remained quiet, letting the words pour out.

"I kept thinking I missed something. That there was something more I could've done. I keep replaying it in my head, over and over. Her blood oxygen levels dropping, her gasping for air, the monitors beeping. I was right there, but I couldn't do anything."

She closed her eyes, the weight of the memory almost unbearable. "I told her it was going to be okay, but it wasn't. And I hate myself for lying to her like that. And I do the same thing with so many others now. I just can't tell them that they are going to be dead slowly and helplessly. "

Dr. Parker leaned forward slightly. "Sophie, it's not your fault. You were doing everything you could, both as her nurse and as her friend. And you are doing the same with your patients too, that's being honest." Sophie shook her head, tears slipping down her cheeks now. "But it wasn't enough. I wasn't enough. I just keep thinking that if I had been better, more attentive, more...something, she might still be here." Dr. Parker's voice was steady but full of empathy. "You're carrying an immense amount of guilt, Sophie, but sometimes even the best care, even all the love in the world, can't change the outcome. You were there for Emily in every way possible. Sometimes, we can't save the ones we love, and that's the hardest thing to accept."

Sophie let out a shaky breath, the tears coming freely now. "I just… I miss my own self so much. And I keep thinking I failed in life."

"You didn't fail, you were there when.." Dr. Parker said softly. "Emily was facing a battle that no amount of care could have won. What you gave her was love, presence, and support in her final moments, and that is invaluable."

The room fell into a quiet stillness, broken only by Sophie's soft sobs. It was the first time she had truly let herself grieve, to feel the weight of losing Emily not just as a nurse, but as her friend. Slowly, through these therapy sessions, Sophie was beginning to confront the truth—that no amount of medical expertise or friendship could have changed Emily's fate. But what she gave Emily in those final moments—the care, the comfort, the companionship—mattered more than she could have realized. As she wiped her tears, Sophie felt a small shift inside her. The grief was still there, sharp and painful, but the crushing guilt that had shadowed her for so long was beginning to loosen its grip. It was the start of a new chapter in her healing, one where she could begin to forgive herself. It's not her fault that she can't stop peoples from dying.

…

Sophie stood frozen, staring at Emily's half-open bag of protest signs and some cloths. It had been taped and left tucked in the corner of her room since she cleaned the room but never opened it, never got the time for it herself, almost forgotten amidst the whirlwind running around, machines, and endless medications.

Sophie kneeled down beside the box, her heart already sinking. She had been avoiding this moment for as long as she could, too focused to confront the lingering feeling that something was wrong. Upon Dr. Parker's advice, today's the day. As she reached inside, her fingers brushed against the familiar crinkling of unopened packages along with protest signs, her makeup kit and some cloths. Prescription bottles. None of it empty.

Sophie pulled them out, her eyes scanning the labels—medications Emily had been prescribed months ago before her passing. Inhalers, steroids, pain relief— all unopened, unused. Her throat tightened, and she felt a wave of disbelief wash over her.

"No..." Sophie whispered, her voice barely audible in the quiet room.

Emily had refused certain treatments before, but Sophie never thought she'd go as far as to hide her prescriptions. There had been arguments about painkillers, oxygen therapy, even intubation. Emily, ever the fighter, always insisted she didn't want to be "drugged up" or "trapped by machines." But Sophie had pushed, pleaded, and convinced her, believing they could prolong her life if only she followed the treatment plan. But this—this hidden bag of unfilled prescriptions felt like betrayal. A silent decision Emily had made without telling her.

Sophie's hand trembled as she turned the bottles over, seeing the prescribed dates on them, realizing how long it had been since Emily had given up on the medications. She had known all along, Sophie realized with a sharp pain in her chest. Emily had known how much time she had left, and she had chosen to live on her own terms. Didn't she wanted to live more? Had she lost the battle the moment diagnosis came?

Sophie ran to the hospital and collapsed into the hospital chair, clutching the prescriptions in her hands. She wanted to check with doctors if they're still usable for someone else battling the similar condition but she just couldn't move. Tears began to flow freely, her chest heaving with sobs she had been holding in for weeks. She had been Emily's nurse, her best friend. She should have noticed. She should have seen the signs. But she was so focused on keeping Emily alive that she missed the fact that Emily had stopped trying.

It all became too much— the machines beeping softly in the background, the smell of antiseptic, the stark whiteness of the walls. Everything around her blurred as the weight of her guilt and grief crashed down. Sophie bent over, her face buried in her hands, sobbing uncontrollably. She had spent every waking moment by Emily's side, trying to manage her treatments, adjusting her oxygen levels, trying to give her more time. And yet, Emily had silently decided that time didn't matter anymore.

The door opened softly, and one of the other nurses peeked inside. "Sophie? Are you okay?" But Sophie couldn't answer. She couldn't even lift her head. The pressure of her failure, her inability to save Emily, crushed her. She had thought they were fighting together, but all this time, Emily had already accepted the inevitable. She never took medicines she was supposed to take.

Chapter 6: Love in the Time

Jack and Amelia's late-night talks at *The Tipsy Oak* shifted from their usual playful banter to deeper, more serious conversations. As the bar emptied and the world quieted, they found solace in each other's company. Amelia, with her sharp wit and no-nonsense demeanour, became the one person who could break through Jack's emotional walls.

One night, as they sat at the bar after closing, Jack stared into his whiskey glass, swirling the amber liquid absentmindedly. “I feel like… no matter what I do, I’m betraying what I use to be,” he muttered. His voice was low, the guilt weighing heavily on him. It was the first time he’d admitted it out loud.

Amelia, wiping down the bar counter, glanced at him. “How?” she asked, her tone direct but not unkind. “By living?”

Jack shrugged, his shoulders hunched. “By moving on. By… feeling anything good. I wasn’t there for good, not when it counted. I let myself down. And now… I don’t know how to be here without feeling like I’m spitting on that memory.”

Amelia set down her rag and leaned on the bar, looking at him with piercing eyes. “You think anyone would want you to live like this? To drown yourself in liquor?”

He winced, her words cutting straight to his core. “I don’t know. Maybe I would. Maybe no one wouldn’t. But I am not the person I should’ve been.”

Amelia didn’t sugarcoat things. “You weren’t perfect, Jack. But no one is, it’s alright, you can’t go back and relive the past all over again to make it right, whatever is left ahead, you can make it right, that’s saving yourself from going more wrong. You can’t keep punishing yourself for something you had no control over at some point.” Her voice softened just a little, the tough exterior peeling back. "And feeling something good now? That's not incomplete. That's surviving."

Jack looked at her, his eyes clouded with emotion. He wanted to believe her. He wanted to let go of the burden, to stop feeling like every step he took forward was an affront to his memory. But it wasn't that easy. He had carried this depression for so long that it felt like a part of him.

Amelia's tough love was exactly what he needed—someone who wasn't afraid to call him out but also wasn't going to let him wallow. She was the one person who saw through his façade, who wasn't afraid to push him to confront the darkness inside him. And slowly, over those late-night conversations, something shifted between them. The nights where they laughed over sarcastic comments and joked about bar patrons gave way to more intimate moments. They began talking about life, grief, and the weight of moving on. Amelia shared stories about her own losses, her rough upbringing, and how she learned to keep going. Jack found himself leaning on her more, seeking her out after long days, craving her presence in a way he hadn't with anyone else since Liam. It wasn't until one night, after a particularly raw conversation, that something between them snapped. The tension that had been building finally came to a head. Amelia reached out, placing her hand on his arm. Jack looked up, and for the first time in a long while, he allowed himself to feel something other than pain. Their kiss was hesitant at first, a mix of confusion, guilt, and longing. But as they pulled away, Jack felt a rush of emotions—relief, desire, and, buried deep beneath it all, fear. He wanted to be close to Amelia, to let her in, but the shadow of his depression still loomed large.

Over the next few weeks, their relationship deepened, becoming romantic in a way neither of them had planned.

Jack found comfort in Amelia's arms, but every time they kissed or touched, there was a part of him that couldn't shake the feeling that he was betraying her and himself, that this all will fall over and out at some point. It was as if moving on, feeling happiness, was a betrayal of the past. He struggled with it silently, not wanting to burden Amelia with his internal battle, but the weight of it was ever-present. Amelia, for her part, noticed. She could see the way Jack would sometimes pull back, the way his smiles didn't quite reach his eyes when they were together. One night, as they lay side by side, she turned to him and said softly, "You don't have to feel guilty for feeling something, Jack."

"I don't know how not to," he admitted, his voice barely above a whisper.

Amelia sighed, brushing her fingers through his hair. "Depression doesn't go away just because you start to live again. It's not one or the other. You can carry your good self with you, and still have room for something new." Jack swallowed, her words settling heavily in his chest. He knew she was right, but it didn't make it easier. He wanted to move forward, to let himself care for Amelia the way he was starting to, but that never ending circle of his own shadows was always there, like a skin he couldn't shake.

Their relationship grew slowly, with Jack learning to let Amelia in little by little. She was patient, never pushing him too far, but always there, challenging him when he needed it. Jack's heart was still heavy with depression, but with Amelia, he began to see glimpses of a future that wasn't completely dark—a future where he could live without feeling like he was living than just existing. But even as their romance blossomed, Jack knew that healing wasn't linear. He would still have to face his demons, to come to terms with the fact that moving on didn't mean forgetting. And with Amelia by his side, maybe—just maybe—he could learn to live with the weight of his past while still allowing himself to embrace the possibility of a future.

...

As Sophie's ALS awareness project began to gain traction, she found herself spending more time with Nate, not just as a colleague, but as a trusted confidant. Together, they worked tirelessly to design pamphlets, organize fundraising walks, and raise awareness for a cause that had become deeply personal to Sophie after losing Emily. Nate's enthusiasm and support were constant, but it was his emotional steadiness that became her lifeline. Their partnership, which had initially been strictly professional, began to evolve. Late nights at the hospital planning the project turned into conversations about life, grief, and their shared experiences. Nate was always quick with a joke, his lighthearted nature offering a momentary escape from the heavy emotional toll Sophie carried. He had a way of making her smile—something she hadn't done much with anyone since Emily's passing.

One evening, after another long planning session, Nate and Sophie sat on a bench outside the hospital. The cool night air provided a brief respite from the intensity of the day. Nate leaned back, glancing over at Sophie, who was lost in thought, her mind likely replaying memories of Emily.

"You know," Nate said, his voice soft, "you're doing an incredible thing here, Soph. Emily would be proud."

Sophie's chest tightened. Nate's words were comforting, but they also brought back the raw pain she tried so hard to bury. "I just... I couldn't save her, Nate," she whispered, her voice barely audible. "I was her nurse. Her friend. And I couldn't do anything. My mistake was I trusted her with medicines and being with herself. She didn't took the medicines and then one night cut off the oxygen tank's tube."

Nate turned to face her, his expression filled with understanding. "You did everything you could, Sophie. Some things... they're out of our control, no matter how much we want to change them."

Sophie's eyes filled with tears, and for the first time, she let them fall in front of Nate. He didn't rush to comfort her with words. Instead, he sat with her in the silence, letting her feel the weight of her grief.

As the days passed, their connection deepened. Nate was her rock—steady, calm, and always there when she needed someone to lean on. He seemed to understand her in ways that others didn't, never pushing her beyond what she was ready to give but always making sure she knew he was there. But as their bond grew stronger, Sophie felt a new kind of fear creep in. The idea of letting someone in, of caring for someone the way she was beginning to care for Nate, terrified her. What if she lost him too? What if she opened herself up, only for everything to fall apart again?

One evening, after a long day of work, Nate offered to walk Sophie home. They strolled through the quiet streets of New York, the city lights flickering around them. There was an unspoken tension in the air, the kind that comes when feelings are on the verge of being acknowledged but held back by fear.

As they reached Sophie's apartment, she hesitated before turning to Nate. "Thank you for everything," she said quietly.

"I don't know how I would've gotten through all of this without you." Nate smiled, but there was a gentleness in his eyes. "I'll always be here, Sophie. You know that."

The sincerity in his voice made Sophie's heart ache. She wanted to tell him how much he meant to her, how his presence had helped her survive the darkest moments. But the fear of losing him, of opening herself up to another potential heartbreak, held her back.

"I'm not sure I'm ready for..." Sophie trailed off, unsure of how to finish the sentence. She didn't even know what she was trying to say.

Nate nodded, his expression understanding. "I get it, Soph. You don't have to explain. I'm not going anywhere, but I also won't push you for more than what you're ready to give."

His words gave her a sense of relief and yet stirred something deep within her. Nate understood her grief, her fear, and he respected her need for space. But as much as she appreciated his patience, part of her longed to take the leap and let him in fully.

Over time, their relationship became a delicate balance. They were close, emotionally and physically, but Sophie kept an invisible wall up—one that Nate never tried to push through. He gave her the space to process her emotions, but his presence was unwavering.

As they worked on the ALS project, Nate's gentle teasing and support helped Sophie rediscover parts of herself that she thought had been lost in her duty. She smiled more, laughed more, and even began to hope again. But the fear of losing someone she cared about lingered like a shadow, reminding her of the fragility of life. And yet, every time Nate looked at her with those patient, kind eyes, Sophie felt a flicker of something more. Something she was terrified to acknowledge but couldn't ignore. It was only a matter of time before she would have to decide whether to keep running from her fear or let herself embrace the possibility of love amidst the chaos.

Chapter 7: Honouring the Fallen

As Jack approaches the end of his grief therapy program, something begins to shift inside him. The sessions and his work with teens at the community centre start to open a path forward. Despite his resistance, Jack begins to realize that healing doesn't mean forgetting — it means finding ways to live alongside the sadness.

Jack fully commits to working with grieving teens at the local community centre, where he partners with Mason to develop an art therapy program. What had started as a reluctant agreement to help out at grief workshops has now blossomed into a sense of purpose. The teens have become his way of channeling his pain into something productive. Watching them use art to express their feelings—whether it's through painting, writing, or music—reminds Jack of Liam's passion for creativity and how it had always been Liam's outlet.

Mason, with his oddball jokes and upbeat energy, proves to be an essential part of Jack's journey. After that fateful encounter at The Green Bean, Mason had stuck by Jack's side, gently nudging him to confront his future. Now, the two of them work side by side, helping teens process their grief through art and creativity. One afternoon, Jack watches a group of teens painting in the community centre's art room. They're quiet, absorbed in their work, and Jack finds himself reflecting on his own journey. Mason walks over, carrying a tray of coffee, and sits down next to Jack.

"You're thinking too hard, man," Mason says with a grin, handing Jack a cup.

Jack smirks, taking a sip. "I think that's your job now, Mason. You're the one always pulling me out of my head."

Mason laughs. "True, true. But seriously, look at what we've done here. These kids, they're getting through it. You're getting through it."

Jack nods, his eyes drifting back to the teens. "Yeah, I guess." But as much as Jack has found purpose in this work, he knows that his journey isn't over. Mason seems to sense this, as he always does. "You know, it's okay to let go of the dark stuff, Jack."

Jack looks over at him, feeling a mix of gratitude and frustration. "I know that. I just… It's not that easy."

Mason nods, his expression softening. "No, it's not. But maybe this—what we're doing—it's enough. You're honouring this blessed life by helping these kids."

Jack doesn't respond right away. Instead, he watches one of the teens pick up a guitar and start strumming, the chords echoing softly through the room. Music had always been Liam's way of connecting with the world, and seeing this teen use it as an outlet brings a bittersweet smile to Jack's face.

“I think you’re right,” Jack finally says, his voice quiet. “It’s not easy, but… maybe this is enough.”

As the art therapy program grows, so does Jack. He still has his moments of doubt, and there are days when the depression feels as dark as it did in the beginning. But now, he has a way of channeling it into something meaningful, something that can help others the way Liam had helped him in navigating life.

Mason continues to be a grounding presence in Jack’s life, helping him navigate the difficult balance of healing while holding onto the memories that matter. Together, they build something that gives grieving and anxious teens a voice, a way to express their emotions when words fail. Though Jack’s internal conflict remains—a constant push and pull between depression and light and healing—he’s no longer running from it. He’s learning to live with it, to accept that grief will always be part of his story. But now, instead of letting it consume him, he’s finding ways to use it as fuel for something greater. The journey isn’t over, but for the first time in a long while, Jack feels like he’s on the right path, in the lives he’s helping to change.

…

Sophie pours every ounce of her energy into organizing the biggest event she’s ever handled: a massive fundraiser for ALS and COPD awareness. It’s not just about raising money; it’s about honouring Emily and the countless others who’ve struggled with these diseases. The event is set to be held at Brighton University, a place rich with memories of Emily, making the occasion both poignant and overwhelming for Sophie.

The weeks leading up to the event are a whirlwind. Sophie juggles her shifts at St. Luke's Medical Center with late-night calls to sponsors, planning committees, and volunteers. Doctors from across the city are eager to contribute, including Dr. Richards and Dr. Sara Thompson, who've both been involved in Emily's care. Sophie's colleague, Nate, is by her side throughout the process, acting as her sounding board and emotional support when the stress begins to take its toll.

As the event day draws nearer, Sophie begins to feel the weight of it all. It's more than just a logistical challenge—it's deeply personal. Every time she finalizes a speech or confirms a guest, she thinks of Emily. Memories of Emily's final days, her protests, her quiet strength, and even the inhalers she didn't use flood Sophie's mind, leaving her torn between guilt and determination.

On the morning of the event, the auditorium at Brighton is buzzing with activity. Rows of chairs are set up, the stage is adorned with banners highlighting ALS and COPD awareness, and tables are filled with pamphlets and information about the diseases. Volunteers usher in patients, survivors, and their families, while medical professionals prepare their presentations.

Sophie stands at the centre of it all, both overwhelmed and empowered. It's the biggest moment of her career and her life. She's organized panels featuring doctors discussing new treatments, survivors sharing their journeys, and researchers talking about the future of care for these devastating diseases. But the heart of the event comes during Sophie's speech, which she's rewritten a dozen times in the days leading up to the event. When she finally steps up to the podium, her hands tremble slightly as she looks out into the sea of faces—doctors she respects, patients she cares for, friends and strangers who've come to support the cause. And then, she spots Emily's parents sitting in the front row, clutching each other's hands.

Her voice cracks at first, but she pushes through. Sophie talks about Emily—not just as a patient, but as a friend. She tells the crowd about Emily's fiery passion for environmental justice, her refusal to back down from a fight, and how her strength in the face of her disease left an indelible mark on everyone who knew her. She also talks about Liam, his humour in the darkest moments, and the way he made the world feel a little less heavy.

As she continues, Sophie's voice grows stronger. She shares her guilt, admitting that she's spent months reviewing Emily's medical records, wondering if she missed something, if she could have done more. But she tells the crowd that the purpose of this event isn't to dwell on the "what ifs." It's to make sure that no one faces what Emily and so many others did without support, without hope. They shouldn't consider these diseases as fatal, the moment we do that, there itself we loose the battle. Then we don't want to waste any more of our resources for the inevitable. Hope shall always remain a priority and that no disease is fatal—should be the way of approach and the attitude.

The room is silent by the time she finishes, the weight of her words hanging in the air. As she steps back from the podium, the audience erupts into applause, and tears fill her eyes. For the first time, Sophie feels like she's truly honouring Emily's legacy, turning her grief into something powerful, something that can make a difference.

The ALS and COPD awareness event is packed with informative and emotional moments, each segment designed to not only educate but also inspire action. The auditorium at Brighton University fills with medical professionals, survivors, patients, and supporters, all eager to learn and honour the cause.

Dr. Thompson, a senior physician and leading pulmonologist, kicks off the medical discussions with a compelling speech on the latest advancements in COPD treatments. She delves into new inhalers, long-acting bronchodilators, and cutting-edge combination therapies that have shown promising results in improving lung function and quality of life. Her presentation includes:

- Inhaled corticosteroids for patients with frequent exacerbations, helping reduce inflammation and prevent worsening symptoms.
- Triple therapy combining inhaled corticosteroids, bronchodilators, and muscarinic antagonists, which has become the gold standard in severe cases.
- New non-invasive ventilation techniques aimed at supporting patients with severe lung disease, allowing them to breathe easier without resorting to invasive procedures.

As Dr. Sara talks, a slideshow of patient success stories plays behind him, offering real-world examples of how these treatments are changing lives. Her speech emphasizes the importance of early intervention, urging primary care physicians and pulmonologists to work together to diagnose COPD in its earliest stages before irreversible lung damage occurs.

Following her speech, a panel of experts takes the stage to discuss the critical need for early diagnosis of COPD and ALS. The panel Dr. Richard, the neurologist, and patient advocates who stress the importance of:

- Recognizing early symptoms: Chronic coughing, shortness of breath, and difficulty breathing often go unnoticed or are dismissed as minor issues, delaying life-saving treatments.
- Routine screening: For at-risk populations, including smokers and those with a family history of respiratory or neurodegenerative diseases, early testing can make all the difference.
- Patient education: Empowering patients to seek help at the first sign of symptoms, rather than waiting until the disease has progressed to an advanced stage.

The conversation shifts to a personal level when one of the panelists, a nurse who lost her father to ALS, shares the emotional toll that delayed diagnosis took on her family. Her voice cracks as she speaks about how her father's symptoms were initially dismissed, leading to a later diagnosis when little could be done. This transitions into the next segment, where Sophie takes the stage again.

As the spotlight shifts to Sophie, the room falls silent. She steps up to the podium, gripping the edges as she prepares to speak. The words she's rehearsed in her mind for weeks now feel heavy as she begins to tell Emily's story.

Sophie starts by sharing who Emily was before the illness took over—her passion for environmental justice, her fierce determination, and her unyielding strength. Then, Sophie talks about the first signs of Emily's COPD, and how, at first, Emily dismissed them, not wanting to believe that her body was failing her. Sophie recounts the progression of Emily's disease:

- The constant breathlessness that worsened over time.
- The oxygen machines that soon became Emily's constant companions.

- The heartbreaking moment when Emily, despite being a fighter, began to refuse certain treatments because she couldn't bear the endless cycle of hospitalizations.

Tears fill Sophie's eyes as she talks about the final days, Emily's refusal to accept certain treatments, and how Sophie, as both a nurse and a friend, felt utterly helpless. She shares the guilt she's carried—about whether she could have done more, said something different, or acted faster. The most heart-wrenching moment comes when Sophie reveals how she found Emily's unfilled prescriptions in her bag after she passed, a discovery that shattered her emotionally.

The crowd sits in silence, many wiping away tears, as Sophie finishes with a powerful statement: "This event isn't about reliving the pain. It's about making sure that no one, no patient or family, has to go through this alone. It's about ensuring that we honour those we've lost by fighting harder for the next person diagnosed."

As Sophie steps down from the podium, the audience erupts into a standing ovation again. The event has not only raised awareness but has deeply touched everyone present, leaving an indelible mark on their hearts.

The event finalises with a fundraising walk around the university campus. Survivors, patients, doctors, and supporters all come together, walking in solidarity for the cause. Sophie walks alongside Nate, who smiles at her, proud of the monumental task she's accomplished. There's a quiet understanding between them, a recognition that Sophie has finally begun to heal, even though the scars of her loss will always remain. By the end of the day, Sophie is exhausted but fulfilled. The fundraiser is a huge success, raising significant funds for ALS and COPD research and bringing attention to the diseases in a way that feels meaningful. As she sits down to rest, Nate hands her a bottle of water and gives her a reassuring squeeze on the shoulder.

“You did it, Soph,” he says softly. “Emily would be proud. And I am too…so you should be you know.”

Sophie nods, wiping away a stray tear. “I hope so,” she replies, her voice barely a whisper. In that moment, surrounded by the people she’s worked so hard to bring together, Sophie realizes that this event isn’t just about ALS or COPD—it’s about love, loss, and the connections that bind people together. It’s about remembering, healing, and finding hope in the midst of grief and moments of indecision. The event concludes with a call to action. Participants are encouraged to donate, support ALS and COPD research, and raise awareness in their communities. Doctors are urged to prioritize early diagnosis, and patients are reminded that they are not alone in their fight. The atmosphere is filled with both somber reflection and a renewed sense of purpose as the crowd leaves, inspired to take action in memory of Emily, Liam and countless others who have faced these devastating diseases.

Chapter 8: Finding Peace

After years of internal struggle and emotional avoidance, Jack experiences a breakthrough at the community centre. One afternoon, he watches a young musician, a teen who reminds him of Liam in his early days, practicing in the corner with a worn-out guitar. The boy's passion for music is palpable, but his instrument is barely holding together, its strings frayed, and the sound is distorted.

Jack quietly observes, emotions stirring within him. Liam's old guitar has been sitting in his apartment for years, untouched, a constant reminder of the life Liam never got to fully live. Jack had clung to it, afraid that letting it go would be betraying his friend. But now, in this moment, he realizes that holding onto it wasn't keeping Liam alive—it was keeping him from healing.

After the teen finishes playing, Jack approaches him, hesitating for a second before saying, "Wait here." He returns hours later, carrying Liam's prized guitar. The boy's eyes widen in disbelief as Jack holds it out to him.

"This belonged to someone who loved music as much as you do," Jack says, his voice thick with emotion. "He didn't get to play it for as long as he should've. But I think he'd want you to have it. And you know what..this belonged to Elvis once."

The boy's hands tremble as he takes the guitar, looking up at Jack with gratitude. As Jack watches him strum the first few chords, a sense of peace washes over him. For the first time in years, he feels like he's truly honoured Liam's memory by passing on the gift of music to someone else. It's a quiet but powerful release, the weight of guilt he's carried slowly lifting.

…

The culmination of Sophie's healing comes at another closing ceremony of her ALS and COPD awareness project. The room is filled with doctors, patients, and supporters, but for Sophie, it's not just a professional achievement—it's a deeply personal one. Standing before the crowd, she takes a deep breath, knowing this moment is for everyone.

She begins her speech by thanking everyone who helped make the event possible, but then shifts into sharing what this project means to her on a personal level. Sophie speaks about the heartache of losing Emily, not just as a patient, but as her best friend. She opens up about the guilt she carried for months, constantly questioning whether she could have done more.

"Emily was a force of nature," Sophie says, her voice steady but emotional. "She fought every battle like it was her last, and she didn't back down—not even when her body started to. Losing her was the hardest thing I've ever had to face. For a long time, I felt like I wasn't doing enough to honour her memory. But standing here, seeing all of you fight for the same cause that took her from us, I realize now—I am keeping her legacy alive. We all are."

The crowd is silent, hanging on every word as Sophie continues, her voice growing stronger. "This isn't just about raising awareness or funds. This is about ensuring that people like Emily and Liam don't face these battles alone. It's about giving them hope, dignity, and a fighting chance. And I know that's what every one of them would want. Til date I've came across hundreds of such nice hearts who got too little time on their hands and that too very painful. It comes as shock to your system, but if we raise awareness about it and be there for them, they wouldn't feel as much left out."

When she finishes, the room erupts in applause, but it's more than just applause—it's recognition, not only of the work Sophie has done but also of the healing she's achieved. As the event draws to a close, Sophie stands on the stage, looking out at the crowd. She feels a sense of peace she hasn't felt in a long time. Jack, standing in the back of the room, meets her gaze. They exchange a nod, an unspoken understanding passing between them. They have both faced their grief, and though they will never forget Liam and Emily, they have found a way to live with their loss, to carry it with them without being weighed down by it. For the first time in what feels like forever, Sophie and Jack both know they're going to be okay. Not because the pain is gone, but because they've found purpose in it. They've found a way to move forward, carrying the legacies of their friends with them—always. As the event winds down, Jack and Sophie slip outside for a moment of quiet under the stars. The night is cool, a welcome contrast to the emotional weight of the day. They sit on the steps outside the venue, shoulders lightly brushing, both lost in their own thoughts. It's a reflective, almost solemn moment, as they take in what they've just been through. Sophie feels blessed to have Jack back. It took time but better late than never.

Suddenly, Mason, having appeared out of nowhere as he often does, plops down next to them. "Well, look at you two," he says, his voice dripping with mock seriousness. "Who knew the tearful speeches would be so... *waterproof.*"

Jack smirks, wiping his face. "What are you talking about? You were crying harder than anyone."

Mason clutches his chest dramatically. "Excuse me, that was *acting*. I was channeling my inner Oscar-worthy performance. Plus, someone had to outdo your 'tragic bartender guy' vibe."

Sophie, trying to hold back a laugh, snorts. "Yeah, sure, Mason. We all believed it."

Mason leans back, putting his hands behind his head, gazing up at the sky. "All I'm saying is, if Liam were here, he would've made some terrible joke about how all that crying just messed up his hair."

Jack chuckles, the familiar, dry sound bringing warmth to the air. "He really would have."

"Yeah, something like, 'What, I die, and now you two turn into a pair of wet blankets?'" Mason continues, earning a full laugh from Sophie.

Jack shakes his head, unable to stop the smile spreading across his face. "Sounds about right." They sit there for a few more minutes, the stars above twinkling brightly, the heaviness of the day easing just a bit with Mason's humour. It's the kind of irreverence Liam would have loved, the sort of joke that breaks through the weight of everything and brings back memories of simpler, more carefree days. Jack and Sophie sit side by side, the cool evening air settling around them, a quiet contrast to the emotional turbulence of the day. The weight of their grief doesn't feel as suffocating anymore, and for the first time in what feels like forever, they're both at peace with the loss they've carried. There's no need for words in this moment—they've said all they needed to during the event.

Jack glances over at Sophie, and there's a shared understanding in her soft smile. It's the same kind of silent, unspoken connection they've always had, but now it feels different—lighter, clearer. Their grief isn't gone, but it no longer defines them.

Sophie exhales, her gaze drifting up toward the stars. She's finally ready to move forward, knowing that Emily's memory will live on, not just in the speeches she gave today but in the small, everyday ways she continues to make a difference. The fundraising, the awareness projects—each is a way to honour Emily's legacy, but it's also for herself, a way to find healing. Beside her, Jack stretches out his legs, leaning back with a sigh. He feels a similar calmness wash over him. He thinks about Liam's guitar now resting in the hands of a young musician, and for once, it feels right. He'll always miss Liam, but instead of drowning in guilt, Jack's now focused on how he can carry his friend's spirit with him, through the teens he helps and his own life he's rebuilding. They sit quietly, the laughter from earlier fading into the distance, as the stars twinkle softly above them. Their memories—of Evan, of Liam, of Emily—still linger, but now, they live on through Jack and Sophie's actions, through their choices to face the future with strength, love, and hope.

***Breathe Until We Can't* Series**

Part - 4 "Where We Belong"

PREFACE

As I sit down to write this preface for Part 4 of our journey, I'm struck by the profound and intricate tapestry of grief, healing, and love that unfolds within these pages. Their grief was palpable, raw, and unyielding. This next chapter takes us into the realm of life beyond loss—a life where memories are cherished, yet the shadows of the past linger as constant companions. Here, we explore the delicate balance between honouring those we've lost and daring to embrace the beauty of new beginnings.

Writing this section challenged me to confront the complexities of moving forward after heartbreak. Jack and Sophie each embark on their unique journeys of healing, navigating the tumultuous waters of grief while slowly finding solace in their careers, friendships, and newfound relationships. Their stories remind us that while grief is a deeply personal experience, it does not have to be faced alone. The bonds we form with others—whether through love, friendship, or shared pain—can illuminate the path to healing.

As their lives intertwine with new characters and experiences, I hope readers will find themselves laughing amid tears, smiling through sadness, and ultimately rooting for Jack and Sophie to find their way back to joy. There is a universal truth in their struggles—a reminder that while loss can reshape us, it does not have to define us. This story is also a tribute to the resilience of the human spirit. It speaks to the power of connection and the importance of taking those small, sometimes hesitant steps toward healing. It's a celebration of life, love, and the enduring legacies of those we've lost.

As you embark on this next chapter with Jack and Sophie, I invite you to reflect on your own journeys of grief and healing. May their experiences resonate with you, and may you find solace in the knowledge that while the past may leave its mark, the future still holds the promise of love and connection.

Thank you for joining me once again on this emotional journey. Your presence as a reader is cherished, and I hope these pages bring you as much comfort and understanding as they brought me while writing them.

With heartfelt gratitude,

INDEX

Chapter 1: Life Beyond Loss

Jack has settled into his new job as a social worker, throwing himself into the role with determination. His days are filled with the stories of the kids he's working to help—young people who've been through unimaginable struggles but still manage to crack jokes, roll their eyes, and challenge him in ways he didn't expect. There's a kind of fulfilment in it, a purpose he hasn't felt in a long long time, but no matter how hard he tries, memory lingers like a shadow over every success, in every smile he coaxes from the teens, praying that they should never go through what he went through for no good apparent reason.

In the morning, Jack arrives early at the community centre, the air still crisp as he unlocks the door. He takes a deep breath, reminding himself that today is about them—the kids who need him. But as he pulls out his files and starts prepping for the day's group session, his thoughts inevitably drift to Liam. It's little things that trigger it—a certain song playing on the radio or a guitar riff someone strums in the hallway. Memories flood back uninvited, like Liam sitting on the edge of his bed with his guitar, or their shared late-night talks about dreams, touring, and everything they'd wanted to accomplish.

At lunch, he eats with Mason at the corner café, where they often debrief their day. Mason has a way of lightening things up, making fun of Jack's serious face as he says, "You know, you might actually scare these kids into therapy with that grim look." Jack smirks but doesn't respond. He appreciates Mason's humour, but the weight of his depression absence always creeps in. Even the laughter feels different, tinged with the emptiness left behind.

When Jack leads his grief workshops, he feels the bittersweetness of helping others process the same kind of loss he's grappling with. Sometimes, a kid will say something that hits too close to home—a joke masking pain, a story about a friend they can't forget—and Jack has to pause, swallow the lump in his throat, and push through. He wants to tell them it gets better, but he knows that's not entirely true. The loss doesn't go away; it just changes shape. Liam's memory is always there, sometimes in the way Jack taps a rhythm absentmindedly with his fingers, like the beats Liam used to drum out. Other times, it's in the small moments of quiet after the sessions, when Jack stays behind, cleaning up the chairs or tidying the room. He feels Liam's presence as if his old friend is watching over him, proud but still missed.

At the end of the day, Jack walks home, the city buzzing around him, but inside, it's just him and the echoes of the past. He's doing better—helping people, making a difference—but there's still that ever-present tug in his chest, the part of him that will always belong to Liam. The grief hasn't gone away, but it's no longer all-consuming. Jack's learning to live with it, to carry it with him as he builds something new. But Liam's ghost, in the music, in the laughter, in the quiet moments—it'll never really leave. And Jack's starting to accept that maybe that's okay.

Sophie has poured herself entirely into her ALS and COPD activism shifting her focus from the research of it, as if trying to atone for something she couldn't change. She's the one everyone turns to for guidance, for knowledge, for energy—and for a while, it feels good. She's organizing events, leading panels, writing articles, and networking with other medical professionals. She's become the face of the cause in her community, known for her passion and drive. But beneath the surface, Sophie is fraying.

Her days at St. Luke's Medical Center are exhausting. She spends long hours working with respiratory patients, balancing her activism on the side. The weight of it all is starting to show. When she goes home after her shifts, her apartment feels like a pressure cooker. The framed protest sign of Emily's hangs on her wall, a constant reminder of the friend she couldn't save. Sophie tries to push through, telling herself she's doing this for Emily. She has to be strong. But the cracks are starting to form.

At night, her mind won't let her rest. The same dreams keep haunting her—she's back in the hospital room, watching patients struggle for breath, watching the oxygen levels dip lower and lower on the monitor. She's frozen, unable to do anything. In the dreams, they always slip away. Sophie jolts awake, her heart racing, drenched in sweat. But it's not just the ones already passed now. She dreams of her current patients—Ms. Dawson, Oliver, faces she's seen recently, all looking to her with the same helplessness.

The nightmares don't stop. Sophie hasn't been sleeping well, and it's starting to catch up with her. When she walks into work, her colleagues notice the dark circles under her eyes, her distant stares as she looks over patient charts. She's still efficient, still sharp, but there's a hollowness to her now, like she's running on fumes.

During the day, she pushes herself through patient rounds, checking oxygen saturation levels, adjusting ventilators, monitoring treatments. But she finds herself zoning out, staring too long at a chart or pausing outside a patient's room as memories of Emily flash through her mind. The same helplessness she felt during Emily's final days is creeping back into her work, making her second-guess every diagnosis, every decision. Her activism, once a source of strength, is becoming overwhelming. Sophie spends her lunch breaks working on ALS awareness projects, reaching out to potential donors, setting up meetings for her fundraising events. She's juggling it all, but the stress is relentless. She barely eats, her meals left half-finished as she stares at her laptop, answering emails, her fingers trembling from too much caffeine and too little sleep.

The burnout is slowly taking its toll. She tries to hide it, smiling politely when people thank her for her work, or when a doctor tells her she's doing an incredible job. But inside, Sophie is crumbling. The pressure, the constant reminders of loss—it's all becoming too much. She feels like she's drowning in it, yet she doesn't know how to stop. There's a moment, after a long day, when Sophie is sitting in her car in the hospital parking lot, staring blankly at the dashboard. Her phone buzzes with another email about an ALS event she's organizing. She grips the steering wheel tightly, feeling her chest tighten. For the first time in months, Sophie admits to herself that she can't keep doing this. She's exhausted, scared of losing more people and herself, terrified that the next patient will remind her too much of Emily. She can't breathe. The weight of it is suffocating.

...

The anniversary memorial for Liam and Emily, held at their old college for they were the only students who didn't left their education even after they were diagnosed with the fatal diseases, they choose to continue education despite the hardships, it's an inspiration, it was a bittersweet event for Jack and Sophie. The campus felt familiar yet distant, filled with memories of laughter, late-night study sessions, and carefree moments shared with their lost friends. As they approached the event, the atmosphere buzzed with quiet conversations, the lawn decorated with white flowers, a peaceful tribute to the lives Liam and Emily had touched.

The memorial was held in the university's garden, beneath the tall oak trees where the group sometimes used to hang out between classes. A photo of Liam and Emily stood at the centre, framed by flowers and candles. Jack felt a tightening in his chest as he looked at their smiling faces, a reminder of the vibrant, passionate people they had once been. Sophie stood beside him, silent, her hands fidgeting with the bracelet she always wore—Emily's old charm bracelet, a gift from their freshman year.

The speeches began, with professors, friends, and even family members sharing stories about Liam's music and Emily's environmental activism. The beauty of the words was undeniable, but Jack and Sophie could barely focus on them. Every word felt like a small cut, reopening the wounds they'd worked so hard to heal.

At one point, an old professor shared a memory of Emily leading a protest to save a local park from being demolished. Sophie's throat tightened, the image of Emily standing on the front lines of that fight so vivid in her mind. Jack shifted beside her, his fingers gripping the program in his hand, the paper crinkling under the pressure. He wasn't sure if he could sit through the whole event. Then, the music started—Liam's favourite song, a track from his old band, played softly through the speakers. Jack clenched his jaw, willing himself not to lose it in front of everyone. The memories hit him like a tidal wave—Liam, strumming his guitar in their dorm room, joking about how they'd make it big one day. Jack's hand instinctively went to his pocket, feeling the familiar shape of Liam's guitar pick, which he had carried with him every day since Liam's passing.

Sophie glanced at Jack, seeing the tension in his face. She reached over, lightly touching his arm. "It's okay," she whispered. Jack gave a small nod, though he wasn't sure he believed her. After the speeches, everyone was invited to the garden to light candles in honour of Liam and Emily. Jack and Sophie stood back as others slowly made their way to the centre, unsure if they could handle participating. The idea of publicly mourning felt overwhelming, like they'd be exposed, raw, with nothing to shield them from the intensity of their emotions. But as they watched others—old friends, professors, even strangers—step forward to light candles, something shifted. Jack turned to Sophie. "You want to...?"

Sophie hesitated, then nodded. Together, they walked toward the memorial, picking up two small candles from the table. As they lit the flames, the soft glow illuminated the faces of Liam and Emily in the photos. It was beautiful, but it hurt. The kind of pain that doesn't go away, no matter how much time has passed. Standing there, side by side, Jack and Sophie shared a moment of quiet reflection. The event was emotionally draining, but it was also a reminder of why they continued to carry on Liam and Emily's legacies. As the candles flickered in the evening breeze, Jack slipped the guitar pick back into his pocket, and Sophie wiped a tear from her cheek. They didn't say anything to each other—they didn't need to. The weight of the past few years hung between them, heavy but shared. After the memorial ended, they lingered for a moment, looking at the other attendees slowly dispersing. "Want to grab some coffee before we head back?" Jack finally asked, his voice soft but steady. Sophie nodded, giving him a faint smile. "Yeah. I think I could use that."

...

Jack's emotions around Amelia had become a tangled web of confusion and guilt. On one hand, he found comfort in their late-night talks and the easy way they could just sit in silence, the world around them forgotten. Amelia had become a steady presence in his life, someone who understood his rough edges and didn't push him to open up until he was ready. But every time he felt himself growing closer to her, a wave of guilt crashed over him. Jack would catch himself pulling away when Amelia leaned in for a kiss or made a joke about the future, as if letting himself feel something for her meant betraying their friendship and her future. He knew it was irrational, that he wants her to be happy, to find peace. But that didn't stop the gnawing feeling in his chest that told him he wasn't capable to move on, not yet. Maybe not ever. Amelia, perceptive as always, noticed the hesitation, though she never pressed him about it. She was patient, but Jack knew it wasn't fair to her, not when part of him was still stuck in the past. Still clinging to memories of his depression, still haunted by the thought that moving on meant leaving a piece of his best friend behind.

For Sophie, the weight of everything felt heavier by the day. She had become the go-to person in her circle for support, the strong one who kept moving forward despite the pain that lingered beneath the surface. Her colleagues at the hospital admired her resilience, her dedication to ALS and COPD activism. But none of them saw the cracks forming beneath that façade.

Sophie wished she could tell someone how much she was struggling. She wished she had someone to lean on, someone who could wrap their arms around her and tell her that it was okay to be vulnerable, to not always have it together. But instead, she put on a brave face, pushing herself harder at work, organizing fundraising events, staying late to research medical advancements—anything to keep herself from collapsing under the weight of her own grief. Nate was there, quietly supportive, his gentle teasing offering brief moments of relief. His presence was calming, but Sophie couldn't bring herself to let him in fully. She couldn't risk it. After all, letting someone close again meant the possibility of losing them, and Sophie wasn't sure she could survive another heartbreak like the one she'd experienced with Emily. Still, there were moments—fleeting, delicate moments—when Sophie found herself wanting to lean into Nate's kindness, to let him be the person she confided in. But the fear of losing him, of being hurt again, kept her from crossing that line. So, she kept her distance, remaining emotionally guarded while quietly wishing she had the strength to just let go.

Chapter 2: New Struggles

Sophie first meets Dr. Liam Harp during a medical conference on neurodegenerative diseases at Columbia. He is a tall, poised man in his mid-fifties, with silver hair and sharp eyes that reflect decades of experience in ALS research. His reputation as a leading specialist precedes him—doctors and researchers alike spoke of him with a mix of reverence and awe. When Sophie shakes his hand, his grip is firm, but his expression is warm, immediately putting her at ease. Dr. Harp had heard about Sophie's work in ALS activism and her dedication to patient care at St. Luke's Medical Center. He commends her passion and drive, but as their conversation deepens over coffee, it becomes clear he sees something in her that most people don't.

"I've seen it before," Dr. Harp says, leaning back in his chair. "Young doctors, nurses, activists—they pour everything they have into the cause, especially when it hits close to home. But the truth is, burnout is real, and it doesn't discriminate."

Sophie listens quietly, feeling her chest tighten. She knew where this conversation was headed. It's like he knew her all her life and knows just what she's feeling and going through.

"You can't help anyone if you're running on empty," Dr. Harp continues, his voice calm but firm. "I understand your dedication to ALS, and I respect it. But there's a limit to how much you can give before it starts affecting your own mental health. If you keep pushing like this, Sophie, you're going to burn out, and that won't help anyone. Least of all yourself."

His words hit her harder than she expected. Sophie shifts uncomfortably in her seat, the familiar guilt bubbling to the surface. How could she step back? She had promised herself that she would keep Emily's legacy alive through her activism. She had become a voice for ALS patients and families, and stepping away felt like a betrayal.

"But I owe it to her," Sophie whispers, her voice barely audible. "To Emily. To all the others."

Dr. Harp leans forward, his expression softening. "I know you do. But part of honouring their memory is also taking care of yourself. You can't fight this battle alone, and you certainly can't do it if you're not at your best, physically or mentally."

Sophie's heart pounds in her chest. The weight of her exhaustion, the nightmares, the constant pressure she put on herself—it all came crashing down in that moment. She knew Dr. Harp was right, but the guilt was overwhelming. How could she even begin to pull back when so many people depended on her?

"I'm not telling you to stop," Dr. Harp clarifies. "I'm saying you need to balance your activism with your own well-being. Take a step back, let others help carry the weight. You've done so much already, Sophie, and there's no shame in acknowledging when it's time to take care of yourself."

Sophie nods, though the conflict still rages inside her. She doesn't know if she can. The idea of stepping back, even for a moment, feels like she's letting Emily and herself down. But deep down, Sophie knows Dr. Harp's words are rooted in wisdom. She's been running on fumes for months, and if she keeps going at this pace, she might not be able to help anyone, not even herself.

As their conversation comes to an end, Dr. Harp hands Sophie his card. "If you ever need to talk, or if you're interested in collaborating on ALS research, I'm here. But remember, your mental health is just as important as your work. Don't forget that." Sophie leaves the meeting torn. Guilt weighs heavily on her, but Dr. Harp's words linger in her mind. Maybe it was time to take a step back. But how could she forgive herself if she did?

...

Jack watches Noah across the room during one of their grief therapy sessions at the community centre. Noah is a wiry fifteen-year-old, his expression guarded, arms crossed defensively. His baseball cap is pulled low, shadowing his face, and his posture screams "leave me alone." He hasn't said more than a few words in any session so far, but Jack recognizes the look in his eyes—the same emptiness and frustration Jack has carried since losing Liam, Emily and mainly himself. Jack knows what it feels like to want to shut out the world.

The rest of the group chatters around them, a mixture of teens at different stages of grief, some talking, some staring at the floor. Jack keeps his eyes on Noah, waiting for any opening, any moment to break through. But Noah's resistance is palpable. He stays quiet, avoiding eye contact, playing with the frayed edges of his hoodie.

After the session ends and the others filter out, Jack approaches Noah cautiously. "Hey," Jack says, keeping his tone light. "You sticking around for a bit?"

Noah shrugs, shoving his hands deep into his pockets. He doesn't say a word, but he doesn't leave either. Jack takes that as a small victory.

"You don't have to talk if you don't want to," Jack continues, pulling up a chair beside him. "But I've been where you are. Losing someone—well, it messes you up in ways you can't always explain, right?"

Noah's lips twitch, almost like he's going to say something, but instead, he remains silent. Jack sighs inwardly, knowing he can't push too hard.

"Look, I get it," Jack says, leaning back. "Therapy sucks when you don't want to be here. I didn't want to be here either at first. Didn't want to talk to anyone. Thought I could just drink, sleep it off, and forget everything."

He pauses, gauging Noah's reaction, but the teen is still impassive, his fingers tapping nervously against the side of his chair. Jack knows he has to be careful. Noah isn't going to open up just because Jack tells him he's been through it, too.

"It's hard," Jack admits after a beat of silence. "You think if you start talking about it, the pain will just get worse. Like maybe it'll make it all more real, and you'd rather just keep it locked up."

For the first time, Noah glances at him. It's a quick flicker of eye contact, but it's there.

"I get why you don't want to talk," Jack adds, his voice softer now. "But you're not alone in this. I know it feels like it—trust me, I know—but you're not."

Noah scoffs, the first real sound Jack's heard from him. "Yeah, right," the teen mutters, his voice low and rough.

Jack doesn't push. He lets the silence linger between them for a while longer. He can feel the frustration in Noah, the anger simmering just below the surface. It's the same anger Jack felt after Liam's death in his depression—the feeling of helplessness and being cheated by the world.

"You don't have to trust me," Jack finally says. "But I'm here if you ever want to talk. No pressure. No judgment."

Noah doesn't respond, but Jack catches the briefest glimpse of emotion in his eyes—something raw and vulnerable, even if it's buried beneath layers of resistance. Jack can tell that breaking through to Noah will take time, but he's willing to put in the effort. He sees himself in Noah's anger and pain, and he knows how hard it is to let anyone in. Jack won't force it, but he won't give up either.

"See you next week?" Jack asks as he stands up, giving Noah one last chance to engage.

Noah shrugs again, but this time it's a little less dismissive, a little less cold. Jack takes that as a small step forward, knowing that healing—like everything else—takes time.

...

Sophie's relationship with Nate unfolds quietly, almost in the background of her chaotic life. They see each other every day at St. Luke's Medical Center, exchanging knowing glances during shifts, sharing the occasional coffee in the staff lounge, and working late nights on her ALS awareness project. But despite the growing closeness between them, Sophie feels like she's constantly holding something back, unsure if she can let herself fully fall. It's not that she doesn't trust Nate. In fact, he's one of the few people she can depend on. His calm presence has been a grounding force in the whirlwind of her life, especially as the anniversary of Emily's death approaches. Nate always seems to know when she needs a break, offering her a warm drink or a moment of quiet away from the hectic pace of the hospital. His gentle teasing brings out her rare smiles, though she often wonders how long she can keep her heart guarded.

One evening after an exhausting shift, they find themselves sitting on a bench outside the hospital, watching the sunset cast long shadows across the parking lot. Sophie's shoulders are tense, her mind preoccupied.

"You look like you're about to solve the meaning of life," Nate says, his voice breaking through her thoughts. His tone is light, but there's an underlying concern in his eyes.

Sophie gives him a small smile, the kind that doesn't quite reach her eyes. "Just...thinking."

Nate nods, leaning back against the bench, waiting. He never pressures her to talk, never pries into the things she's not ready to share. But he's always there, always patient.

"I don't know if I can do this," Sophie admits after a long pause, surprising herself with the admission. "Not just this project, but... everything."

Nate doesn't interrupt, giving her the space to continue.

"It feels like I'm waiting for the other shoe to drop. Like if I get too close, if I let myself care too much, I'm just going to lose someone else." Her voice falters, and she hates how vulnerable she feels saying it out loud. She's been holding onto this fear for so long—this constant dread that if she opens up again, the universe will rip something else away from her. Nate turns to her, his expression gentle but serious. "You don't have to rush anything, Sophie. We're not on some timeline."

Sophie sighs, running a hand through her hair. "I know, but... I'm scared, Nate. I'm scared of feeling everything all over again." He reaches out, resting his hand on hers, the gesture simple but filled with meaning. "I get that. And I'm not going anywhere. But you don't have to let all that fear keep you from living."

Sophie closes her eyes for a moment, feeling the weight of his words sink in. She wants to believe him, wants to trust that it's possible to let someone in without the inevitable heartbreak looming over her. But Emily's and her patients death left scars she isn't sure will ever fully heal. Nate doesn't push for more. He just sits with her in the fading light, their hands touching, and for the first time in a while, Sophie lets herself relax just a little. She doesn't have all the answers, and she isn't ready to dive headfirst into something new, but for now, the small comfort of Nate's presence is enough. Their relationship is slow, filled with these quiet, tentative moments. Sophie knows she's holding back, that she's not giving Nate all of herself, but she's not sure she can. Not yet. But maybe, in time, she'll find a way to trust in something more, to let her guard down again. For now, the unspoken connection between them is enough—fragile, but real. And in that moment, sitting in the soft glow of the setting sun, Sophie allows herself to feel something other than fear. Just for a little while.

...

One evening, Sophie invites Nate over for a casual dinner, determined to shift her focus from the heavy weight of her work and the endless thoughts of her life. Cooking, she thinks, might be a good distraction. What she doesn't anticipate is Nate's absolute ineptitude in the kitchen.

"So, have you ever cooked anything besides toast?" Sophie asks, tying her apron and handing Nate a chopping board.

Nate raises an eyebrow, feigning offence. "Excuse me, I'll have you know I make a mean bowl of cereal."

Sophie laughs, shaking her head as she watches him clumsily attempt to chop an onion. "I'm starting to see why you always suggest takeout."

As the evening goes on, things quickly spiral into chaos. Nate's chopping skills are more hazard than help, with onions flying off the board and his knife technique looking like something out of a bad horror movie. Sophie steps in, trying to save what's left of the vegetables, but they're both laughing too hard to focus.

"This is a disaster," Nate admits, holding up a misshapen zucchini with a grin.

"I'm starting to think you're sabotaging dinner just to make me laugh," Sophie says, her laughter still bubbling over as she grabs the zucchini from him. "Step aside, chef. Let the professional handle this." But even Sophie isn't immune to the kitchen chaos. After handing Nate the task of stirring the sauce, she realizes too late that she's left the bread in the oven for far too long. The smell of burnt toast fills the kitchen.

"Oh no!" Sophie gasps, rushing to pull the charred loaf out of the oven. She holds it up like a failed science experiment, glancing at Nate with an exasperated smile. "We're hopeless."

Nate shakes his head, a look of mock seriousness on his face. "You know, I think this might be a sign. We're just meant to eat pizza." Sophie chuckles, wiping her hands on her apron. "You might be right. Cooking is clearly not our strong suit." Despite the kitchen catastrophe, they end up sitting on the floor, surrounded by the remnants of their failed dinner attempt, eating takeout pizza from the box. The disaster has left them in fits of laughter, and for a while, Sophie feels lighter, the burden of her grief momentarily lifted by the playful banter and shared moments of ridiculousness.

"I think I'll stick to the hospital," Nate says, biting into a slice of pizza. "Much safer for everyone involved."

Sophie grins, finally feeling some of the tension leave her body. "Good plan. But next time, I'm teaching you how to boil water. Baby steps." They share a warm, light-hearted moment in the midst of all the emotional heaviness in their lives. And even though the dinner was a complete disaster, it's one of the first times in a long while Sophie finds herself genuinely smiling without the shadow of grief lurking nearby.

Chapter 3: The Weight of the Past

In a quiet moment at the Columbia, Sophie sits across from Dr. Liam Harp, her hands trembling slightly as she pulls out Emily's old medical records. The papers are worn from frequent handling, with highlighted notes and scribbles in the margins from late nights spent obsessively reviewing her friend's case. She's hesitant but knows she needs answers, even if they won't ease her guilt.

"I've been going over Emily's charts," Sophie begins, her voice tight with emotion. "She had stopped using her prescribed inhalers regularly, and I... I should've pushed harder. I keep thinking—what if I missed something? What if there was another treatment? Something that could've..."

Dr. Harp listens intently, his expression calm yet understanding. He's been in these types of conversations before, but he can see how deeply this is affecting Sophie. He gently takes the records from her, skimming through the pages with practiced eyes.

"Sophie," he says after a moment, "Emily's condition had progressed too far. Even if she had followed every prescription to the letter, the outcome wouldn't have changed."

Sophie swallows, feeling her chest tighten. "But the inhalers... if she had kept up with them—" Dr. Harp interrupts gently, but firmly. "Inhalers help manage symptoms, but they're not a cure. With her level of deterioration, there was nothing that could've reversed the damage. Her body was already shutting down. They did everything they could within the limits of medicine."

Sophie's eyes sting as she holds back tears, her gaze fixated on the prescription details she's memorized over and over—the medications Emily should have taken, the unfilled prescriptions she found in Emily's bag after her death.

"I just... I can't stop thinking I could have done more," Sophie whispers, her voice barely audible.

Dr. Harp reaches across the desk, resting a hand on her shoulder. "You were her friend, Sophie, and you did everything you could. Medicine can be unforgiving, but there are things beyond our control. No amount of treatment would have saved her from the inevitable." His words settle heavily over her, offering a small sense of relief, but not entirely washing away the guilt. Sophie knows, deep down, that she will always carry the weight of Emily's loss with her. But Dr. Harp's reassurance provides a glimmer of closure, reminding her that no one could have fought harder than they did, and some battles are simply irreversible. Unwinnable.

...

Jack slings a guitar over his shoulder, its once-polished wood now weathered from years of play. It feels heavier than usual today as he walks through the doors of the community centre, a bittersweet weight he's come to carry with quiet reverence. The building buzzes with the chatter of teens—some familiar, others new. He's still learning their names, their stories, but they all share a thread of loss, much like himself. Today, though, he isn't just here as the "sad bartender guy" anymore.

Mason, already at the centre, catches sight of him and offers a half-smile. "You bring it?" he asks, nodding toward the guitar.

Jack nods, though a hint of hesitation flickers across his face. "Yeah, figured it was time," he mutters, adjusting the strap.

Mason gives him a reassuring nudge. "Good. These kids could use a distraction. Hell, we all could." As the group settles into the room, Jack pulls up a stool and rests the guitar on his knee. His fingers hover over the strings, the familiar feel stirring up memories of late-night jam sessions in their college dorm, Liam grinning, full of life and music. But instead of the familiar ache, Jack finds himself wanting to share that part of his past, not just mourn it.

"Alright, I'm no rock star, I had bought this only so I could have fun with my friend Liam." Jack begins, his voice slightly shaky but laced with humour, "but I'm gonna teach you guys a thing or two about making noise."

The teens laugh, a few skeptical looks exchanged, but they're intrigued. Mason steps up, helping Jack wrangle the kids' attention, and soon enough, they're forming a circle. Jack's fingers begin to strum the opening chords of an old tune. The notes fill the room, soft but full of warmth, and something shifts in the air.

"Who wants to give it a shot?" Jack asks, holding out the guitar. A couple of hands shoot up, and soon the group is taking turns, each plucking out awkward notes and laughing at their failed attempts. But the laughter feels good, light, like a release.

Mason watches from the side, leaning against the wall with his usual smirk. "Not bad, man," he comments when Jack joins him during a break. "You know, I think Liam would've liked this. You, here, passing the torch." Jack exhales slowly, his fingers running over the fretboard. "Yeah. I think so too." Their bond, once centred on grief, now finds a new foundation—one built on shared purpose and the belief that they can do something meaningful with their pain. The music sessions become a staple at the youth centre, offering not just an outlet for the kids, but for Jack too. It's a small step, but each strum of the guitar feels like a step forward, a way to honour his friend while finding his own healing.

The night is chilly as Jack walks up to the small, dimly lit venue where the concert is being held. A group of friends had invited him to the event—a tribute to Liam's old band, with some of their tracks being performed live by a few local musicians who admired them back in college. One of them's Madison. Jack had hesitated at first, unsure if he was ready to confront the flood of memories it would undoubtedly bring. But something in him couldn't say no. Maybe a part of him felt it was time. Inside, the place buzzes with low conversation, the air thick with nostalgia. Photos of Liam's band are pinned up on a small corkboard near the stage—old snapshots from college days, faded with time but full of energy. There's one of Liam, guitar slung across his back, his wild grin lighting up the frame. Jack's stomach tightens as he stares at it. The memories are too vivid—Liam in the spotlight, pouring his soul into his music, the way his laughter echoed backstage after every performance.

He shuffles toward a corner, trying to stay out of view, but several people recognize him immediately. Old college friends and acquaintances approach him, offering warm hugs and bittersweet smiles. "He'd be so proud, man," one of them says, clapping Jack on the back. He forces a smile, nodding, but the words sink into his chest like stones.

The concert begins, the first notes of Liam's most famous track filling the room. The crowd cheers, but Jack's heart races. The song is slower than he remembers, a haunting rendition that reverberates with the absence of its original performer. Every chord feels like a punch to his gut, every lyric a reminder of what's been lost. As the song continues, Jack's emotions churn uncontrollably. He watches as Madison tries to emulate Liam's passion, but it only makes him more aware of how Liam can never take the stage again. The weight of it all becomes unbearable—the laughter, the music, the memories that feel too raw, too real. His breath catches in his throat. Without a word to anyone, Jack stands and quietly makes his way to the exit. His chest feels tight, the cold air outside a sharp contrast to the warmth of the venue. He leans against the brick wall, running his hands through his hair, trying to steady himself. But the sadness, the guilt, it all swells inside him like a storm he can't contain.

Liam's music had always been a part of Jack's life, a source of joy and connection. Now, hearing it feels like an echo of something that's gone forever. Jack pulls his jacket tighter around him, turning away from the venue, unable to bear the weight of it any longer. He leaves without saying goodbye to them, walking into the night, each step heavy with the grief that still clings to him.

...

Jack sits on the porch of Sophie's apartment, the cool night air pressing down on him as he stares out into the darkness. He's been sitting in silence for what feels like hours, the weight of his thoughts suffocating him. Guilt gnaws at his insides, an unshakable presence that has haunted him for years. The concert had stirred something inside him—a deep, painful realization that he couldn't escape. Why was he still here, living, breathing, when Liam, who had so much more to offer the world, was gone?

The door creaks open, and Sophie steps out, wrapping her sweater tighter around her. She quietly takes a seat beside him on the worn-out steps, not saying a word at first. She's learned that sometimes silence speaks louder than any attempt at comforting words.

Finally, Jack breaks the stillness, his voice raw and strained. "I can't shake this feeling, Soph…" His eyes, bloodshot from the unshed tears he's been holding back meet hers, and she can see the depth of his pain.

Sophie sighs softly, looking up at the stars for a moment before answering. "Jack, I've asked myself that same question so many times. I think about the moments we spent together, the plans she had, and I wonder why it all had to go. But… we're not meant to have the answer to that."

"I should've done right," Jack says, his voice shaking. "Life was… was everything. And I just lay there, watching it fade away."

Sophie shifts closer, her hand resting on his arm. "You did everything you could. you knew that. And more than anything, Jack, you wouldn't want this for you. you wouldn't want you drowning in guilt, punishing yourself for something you had no control over. It was just the depression. Many people face it nowadays. Leave it. Don't blame yourself"

Jack clenches his fists, eyes narrowing. "But I am here, Sophie. I'm alive, and sometimes I'm not. How am I supposed to live with that?"

Sophie takes a deep breath, her voice gentle but firm. "By living the life others can't, Jack. By doing what he would have wanted you to do—be happy, find purpose, and remember him without letting his memory break you. He'd hate seeing you like this." Jack shakes his head, a tear finally slipping down his cheek. "I don't know how, Soph. I don't know how to let go of this guilt."

Sophie's grip tightens on his arm, her voice steady. "You don't have to let go of it, not entirely. But you can't let it control you either. Liam lived for the moments that made life worth it—his music, his friends, the stupid jokes he made. He doesn't know the helpless you. He won't like that. Do it for him. He'd want you to find joy again, even if it feels impossible."

Jack wipes at his face, struggling to find his voice. "It feels like I'm betraying him if I'm happy, if I move on."

Sophie shakes her head softly. "Moving on doesn't mean forgetting him. You can honour his memory by living fully, Jack. You think Liam would want you wasting away, feeling like you don't deserve the life you still have?" The words hit him like a punch, and Jack feels something inside him shift. He pictures Liam, grinning like a fool after a late-night jam session, cracking jokes and living without fear. The guilt that had weighed so heavily on him begins to ease, just slightly, as he imagines what Liam would say if he saw him now—how he'd tell Jack to get his act together, to laugh, to live. Jack nods slowly, swallowing hard. "He'd probably tell me I'm being a dumbass." Sophie laughs softly, her eyes misting. "Exactly. He'd want you to live, Jack. Not just for him, but for you." Jack lets out a long breath, feeling the burden of his grief begin to shift ever so slightly. For the first time in a long time, he can see the path forward, however blurry and uncertain. And for the first time, he feels like maybe, just maybe, he can start to live again. He's right, it's only the peoples who've went through the same things as you can understand you enough. And Sophie understood him without him saying much.

Chapter 4: Turning Point

Sophie's calendar is a maze of overlapping appointments, meetings with ALS and COPD foundations, fundraising calls, and shifts at the hospital. Every waking moment is consumed with something—whether it's organizing awareness events, speaking to patients' families, or reviewing treatment plans. Her passion for the causes she holds close is undeniable, but it's beginning to take a toll on her. She hasn't had a full night's sleep in weeks. At the hospital, she takes on extra shifts, convincing herself that the work keeps her mind occupied. But even her colleagues have noticed the dark circles under her eyes and the strain in her voice. On break, Sophie barely eats, more focused on catching up on emails or planning the next fundraiser. She's always moving, always doing—because when she stops, the weight of everything hits her all at once.

Sophie hasn't talked about it with anyone except Dr. Harp, but the nightmares have returned—vivid, unsettling dreams. The emotional strain begins to manifest physically. Her hands tremble as she fills out patient charts, and her usually steady voice wavers when speaking to families. She catches herself zoning out in meetings, overwhelmed by the flood of responsibilities she's piled onto herself.

Nate notices. He's been quietly watching her from the sidelines, worried but unsure of how to approach the subject. One night after a particularly long shift, he catches Sophie as she's getting ready to head out, her bag slung haphazardly over her shoulder.

"Soph, when was the last time you slept for more than three hours?" he asks, concern etched into his features.

She brushes him off with a tired smile. "I'm fine, Nate. There's just a lot going on right now." Nate frowns, not convinced. "You're running yourself into the ground. You can't keep this pace up forever." Sophie shakes her head, avoiding his gaze. "I don't have a choice. There's too much to do. These projects, these patients… they need me."

"And what about you?" Nate's voice softens as he steps closer, his hand gently resting on her arm. "You need you too."

Sophie's chest tightens. She knows he's right, but the guilt she carries is too heavy to let her stop. "I'm fine," she repeats, though the crack in her voice betrays the truth. Nate doesn't push further, but the silence that follows speaks volumes. Sophie heads home, the weight of everything pressing down on her, but even then, she doesn't slow down. She can't. Not when there's so much for her to do.

…

Sophie's newest patient, Alyssa, is a bright, optimistic young woman in her early twenties, recently diagnosed with early-stage COPD. As Sophie reviews Alyssa's medical history, she feels an instant pang of familiarity—Alyssa's situation bears a striking resemblance to Emily's early symptoms. The bond between nurse and patient forms quickly, something Sophie tries to keep professional, but the echoes of her past friendship with Emily are hard to ignore. The initial treatment plan involves standard care—daily bronchodilators to open the airways, corticosteroids to reduce inflammation, and regular check-ins on her oxygen levels. Alyssa is new to the routine, and Sophie spends extra time walking her through each medication, showing her how to properly use the inhalers, and discussing the importance of avoiding respiratory irritants. Sophie's voice is calm and reassuring, but internally, her emotions stir. The conversations with Alyssa soon extend beyond medical advice. During their treatment sessions, Alyssa shares stories about her life—her dreams of finishing college, her passion for photography, and her fears about how the illness might limit her future. Sophie listens intently, offering encouragement, but behind her professional demeanour, she feels the emotional toll growing heavier with each interaction. She couldn't tell her that the time comes sooner than anyone expects.

Every time Sophie takes Alyssa's vitals, she's reminded of the countless times she checked Emily's oxygen levels. She can't shake the image of Emily's final weeks, and the guilt of not being able to save her friend. As Alyssa talks about her future with a hopeful smile, Sophie finds herself haunted by the thought that she may be witnessing another tragedy unfold. The routine checkups continue—spirometry tests to monitor lung function, follow-ups with the pulmonologist, and discussions about lifestyle changes. Sophie ensures Alyssa has access to all the resources she needs—support groups, education on managing flare-ups, and counselling if necessary. But every time Sophie enters the room, a mix of warmth and dread settles in. She grows attached, seeing Alyssa's resilience, her fight to keep her life as normal as possible, and it hits too close to home.

One afternoon, as Sophie adjusts Alyssa's oxygen mask and prepares her for a breathing treatment, Alyssa, sensing Sophie's distant gaze, asks, "Have you ever known someone with this… condition?"

Sophie freezes for a moment, the memories flooding back. She wants to answer honestly but feels the lump in her throat tighten. After a brief pause, she says softly, "Yes. I did."

Alyssa nods, sensing the weight behind Sophie's words. "Did they… make it?"

Sophie forces a smile, her heart heavy with the truth she can't fully share. "They fought really hard." The interaction leaves Sophie emotionally drained. Every time she sees Alyssa, she's reminded of Emily's struggle, and it becomes harder to separate her personal grief from her professional role. She stays later at the hospital after her shifts, pouring over Alyssa's charts, checking every possible detail—lung capacity, oxygen saturation, even her dietary intake—determined not to miss anything this time, not like with Emily. But the bond she's forming with Alyssa isn't just medical anymore. It's personal. And with every step forward in Alyssa's treatment, Sophie can't help but feel the weight of the past creeping in, making it harder to keep her emotions at bay.

…

During one of their sessions at the youth centre, Jack sits across from Noah, the quiet teenager who's been resistant to every form of therapy up to this point. Jack had tried everything—talking, listening, even bringing up music—but nothing seemed to reach Noah. Today, however, Jack had a different idea. He slid a notebook and a pen across the table to Noah. "I want you to write a letter to your parents."

Noah stared at the paper as if it were a foreign object. "What's the point?" he muttered, shrugging as he avoided eye contact.

Jack leaned forward, his tone gentle but firm. "You never got to say goodbye. Maybe this will help."

Noah's hands remained in his lap, fingers twitching, his jaw clenched. Jack recognized the walls Noah was putting up—he'd done the same with Liam's memory for so long. He knew pushing too hard wouldn't help, so he waited, letting the silence settle between them.

After a long pause, Noah finally reached for the pen, though he didn't write right away. Jack could see the tension in his furrowed brow, the hesitation in his shaking hand. The boy started with a few words, slowly scribbling sentences, his pen occasionally pausing as he wrestled with emotions he wasn't ready to confront.

Jack didn't interrupt. He sat beside Noah, offering quiet support, watching the young boy pour years of bottled-up feelings onto the page. As the minutes passed, Noah's scribbling became more fervent, more emotional. Jack could feel the shift—the walls were cracking, and Noah was finally allowing himself to feel.

When Noah finished, he closed the notebook and sat back, staring at the table. His eyes were red, though he didn't cry. Jack gave him space, letting the weight of what he'd just done settle in.

"How does it feel?" Jack asked quietly, knowing the answer wasn't simple.

Noah shook his head, struggling to find the words. "I... I didn't even know what to say to them. It's... it's like they're still here, you know? But not."

Jack nodded, understanding the sentiment deeply. "That's grief. Sometimes it makes you feel like they're still around, even when they're not. But writing that letter? That's a step forward. It's you saying everything you didn't get to before."

Noah wiped at his eyes, the hardened exterior he'd been keeping up starting to fade. For the first time, Jack saw the vulnerability beneath the surface—the fear, the confusion, the pain of losing his parents so young. It reminded him of his own loss, the grief he still carried over Liam and himself.

"I think they'd be proud of you," Jack added softly. "For still being here. For still fighting, even when it hurts."

Noah didn't respond, but Jack could tell the boy was listening, the words settling somewhere deep inside him. There was a long silence before Noah finally muttered, "Thanks." From that moment on, their sessions changed. Noah began to open up more, and the letter-writing exercise became a turning point in their relationship. Jack could see how much the boy had been holding in, and helping him process it became a personal mission. It wasn't just about therapy anymore—it was about helping Noah find his way through a darkness Jack knew all too well.

Jack's bond with Noah deepened over the weeks. He started bringing more creative exercises into their sessions—journaling, storytelling, even movies and music therapy. Slowly, Noah began to trust him, inch by inch. It became clear to Jack that this wasn't just about Noah—it was about both of them. In helping Noah confront his grief, Jack was starting to confront his own.

...

It was late when Sophie and Nate finally wrapped up the ALS awareness meeting they'd been working on for weeks. The room was quiet now, empty, except for the two of them. Sophie sat on the edge of the table, her legs dangling as she gazed out the window at the night sky, feeling a sense of accomplishment but also a deep exhaustion. Nate was packing up the last of their materials, but he paused when he saw Sophie staring off into space. "You okay?" he asked gently, walking over to her. She didn't answer right away, instead watching the stars twinkle faintly in the distance. It felt like the world had slowed down, leaving just the two of them in this quiet bubble. Sophie turned to Nate, her eyes searching his face, and for the first time in a long while, she felt like she didn't have to carry the weight of everything alone. Nate stepped closer, his hand brushing against hers in a way that felt unintentional, yet deeply intentional at the same time. The warmth of his touch sent a rush of something through Sophie—something she hadn't allowed herself to feel in a long time. Without thinking, she closed the distance between them, her lips meeting his in a gentle kiss. For a moment, everything else fell away. It was just them, the softness of the night, the closeness they had built over months of working together.

Nate responded tenderly, his hand cradling her face, as if he understood the fragility of the moment. Sophie leaned into him, letting herself feel the warmth of being held by someone again, of letting her guard down, even just for a little while. It felt right—but then, all at once, it felt terrifying.

Suddenly, Sophie pulled away, her breath catching in her throat. Panic surged in her chest as reality crashed back in. The vulnerability of it all—the closeness, the intimacy, the possibility of getting hurt—it was too much.

"I—I'm sorry," she stammered, stepping back quickly, creating space between them. Her heart was racing, her mind spiralling with fear. What if she got too close? What if then she lost him?

Nate looked at her, his expression soft, understanding. He didn't push or say anything right away, letting her take the space she needed. "It's okay," he said quietly, his voice gentle. "You don't have to apologize."

Sophie shook her head, feeling the guilt, the fear, all of it swirling inside her. "I can't... I don't think I can do this," she whispered, her voice breaking. "I don't know if I can let someone in like that…I don't feel I'm ready."

Nate's face softened even more, and he took a step forward, but only to meet her eyes, not to close the physical distance. "Sophie, I get it. You've been through so much. I'm not here to rush you or push you into anything. I just... I care about you. And I'm here, whenever you're ready."

His words were like a lifeline, but they also scared her even more. The idea that someone cared so deeply—after everything she'd been through cuz of her duties and because she cared, and the constant fear of losing more people—it was overwhelming. She didn't know if she could trust herself to handle that, to risk it.

Sophie looked away, blinking back the tears that were threatening to spill. "I'm just so scared of losing someone," she admitted, her voice barely above a whisper. "I don't know if I can go through."

Nate nodded, his eyes filled with understanding. "I know," he said softly. "And if you need time, that's okay. I'm not going anywhere. And how will you know that if you don't love me." There was a heavy pause as Sophie wrestled with her emotions, torn between wanting to be close to him and the fear that had been keeping her walled off for so long. She felt Nate's presence beside her, steady and patient, and for the first time in a long time, she allowed herself to believe, even just a little, that maybe she didn't have to face everything on her own. But for now, she wasn't ready. "I just need... I need some time," she whispered, her voice shaky but honest. Nate smiled, though it was a soft, understanding smile, not one of disappointment. "Take all the time you need, Sophie. I'll be here."

Chapter 5: Breaking Point

Sophie had been running on empty for weeks, the weight of her ALS and COPD activism, her shifts at the hospital pulling her in every direction. She felt like she had no choice but to keep going—there was too much at stake, too many people depending on her. But her body had other plans. It happened during one of her afternoon rounds. Sophie was checking on a patient when her vision blurred, and a wave of dizziness hit her like a truck. She gripped the edge of the bed, willing herself to stay upright, but her knees buckled beneath her. The last thing she remembered was the sterile smell of the hospital and the muffled sounds of concern as everything went dark.

When she woke, she was in a hospital bed of her own, the familiar beeping of monitors ringing in her ears. She blinked, disoriented, trying to piece together what had happened. Her eyes slowly adjusted to the soft lighting, and she saw Dr. Richard and Nate standing near the door, their faces etched with worry.

"Sophie," Dr. Richard said, his tone stern but concerned. "You collapsed from exhaustion. You've been pushing yourself too hard."

She tried to sit up, her instinct to dismiss the concern kicking in immediately. "I'm fine. I just need a moment. There's too much to do—"

Nate stepped forward, shaking his head. "No, Sophie. You need to stop. This isn't fine. You've been burning the candle at both ends for too long."

Sophie's heart raced, a mix of guilt and frustration bubbling up inside her. "I can't just stop. There are patients who need me, the ALS awareness projects— If I slow down now, I'll be letting everyone down. I'll be letting *her* down."

Dr. Richard sighed, pulling up a chair next to her bed. His voice softened, but there was a seriousness in his gaze. "Sophie, you're a brilliant nurse, and your work in ALS and COPD activism is admirable. But you can't pour from an empty cup. If you keep this up, you're going to burn out completely—physically and emotionally. You have to take care of yourself first."

Sophie clenched her jaw, the thought of stepping back from her work making her feel like a failure. "But I can't," she whispered, her voice cracking. "If I stop, if I take a break...

what if I let people down? What if I let *the hope* down? That's what had happened with Jack..he took a break and never recovered from it again."

Nate stepped closer, his eyes filled with understanding but firm resolve. "Sophie, Emily wouldn't want this for you. She wouldn't want you running yourself into the ground in her name. You've done so much already. It's okay to take a step back and care for yourself. You're human, and you deserve to heal too."

Tears pricked Sophie's eyes, the exhaustion and emotional strain finally catching up to her. She'd been carrying so much for so long, feeling like it was her responsibility to keep everything together, to keep pushing for Emily, for herself, for the patients who reminded her of her friend. But now, sitting in the hospital bed, her body weak and her mind clouded with fatigue, she realized how close she was to breaking.

Dr. Richard's voice was gentle as he placed a hand on her shoulder. "Taking care of yourself isn't selfish, Sophie. It's necessary. You've been through so much, and you've given so much of yourself. You need time to rest, to heal. That's what Emily would want for you."

Sophie wiped at her eyes, her defences crumbling. She hated feeling weak, hated the idea of needing to step away, but deep down, she knew they were right. She was exhausted—physically, mentally, emotionally. Her body had been screaming for a break for weeks, but she had ignored every sign, convinced that stopping would be a betrayal of the work she'd dedicated herself to. But as she looked up at Nate and Dr. Richard, she felt a sliver of relief. Maybe—just maybe—it was okay to stop. Just for a while. Maybe it didn't mean she was giving up.

Nate knelt beside her, his hand finding hers, giving it a reassuring squeeze. "We'll pick up the slack. You're not alone in this. Take the time you need." Sophie took a deep, shaky breath, the tension she'd been holding onto for so long finally beginning to loosen. It wasn't easy—nothing about this was—but for the first time, she allowed herself to consider the possibility of slowing down, of taking a break. For herself. For the future she was still figuring out how to navigate.

...

Jack and Amelia had been navigating their relationship cautiously, treading lightly around the unspoken tension that had been building for months. Jack could feel it in the way Amelia looked at him when he drifted into silence, lost in thoughts, or when he pulled back emotionally just as they started to get closer. It was a delicate balance—one that Amelia had been more than patient with, but tonight, everything seemed to shift.

They sat across from each other in Jack's own new apartment, the small living room lit by the soft glow of a single lamp. Amelia had come over for what was supposed to be a casual dinner, but the weight in the air was palpable. Jack could feel his chest tighten as he avoided eye contact, playing nervously with the edge of his sleeve. Amelia, ever perceptive, finally broke the silence. "Jack, we need to talk."

Her voice was calm but firm, a clear signal that this conversation had been brewing for a while. Jack looked up, meeting her eyes, and he could see the weariness in them—mixed with a determination that made his stomach knot.

"I know," he said quietly, already bracing himself for what was coming. He had been expecting it, in some ways even dreading it. Amelia had been incredibly understanding of the complexities of his grief, but he also knew there was only so much someone could wait for.

Amelia took a deep breath before speaking again. "I need to know where we stand. I care about you, Jack. A lot. But... it feels like you're always halfway here, like you're still stuck in the past. I get that it's hard, I do, but... I need more. I need you to be fully present with me."

Jack's heart pounded in his chest, and he opened his mouth to respond, but no words came out. He *wanted* to be present with Amelia. He cared about her, loved her even—but the shadow of his own uncertainity lingered over every moment they shared. Every time they got close, every time things felt good, the guilt would creep in, whispering that he didn't deserve to be happy forever, that again he'll get back to addiction and depression and everything will again feel like a prison.

"I... I'm sorry," Jack finally said, his voice hoarse. "It's just... it's not that I don't care about you. I do. It's just—"

Amelia cut him off, her tone gentle but resolute. "It's future. I know." She stood up, pacing a little as she gathered her thoughts. "Jack, I've been patient because I understand grief. I understand how hard it is to be so sure like that. But I can't keep waiting for you to get completely perfect, especially when we are getting older with each passing day. It's a disrespect to time."

Her words hit him like a punch to the gut. Jack leaned forward, resting his elbows on his knees as he buried his face in his hands. She wasn't wrong. He *had* been avoiding dealing with his future.

Amelia crouched down in front of him, her hands gently resting on his knees as she spoke softly. "Be happy. And if I'm not what makes you happy, then I need to know that too."

Jack's throat tightened as he lifted his head, meeting her gaze. "It's not you," he whispered, his voice cracking. "It's me. I just... I don't know how to keep moving now. I feel like if I do, it means something'll go wrong."

Amelia's expression softened, but there was still an edge of frustration there. "You have to let yourself heal first. You can't keep punishing yourself for being alive."

Jack felt tears welling up, and he blinked them away quickly. He hadn't cried like this in front of anyone, not even Sophie. It was as if he'd been holding his grief and guilt so tightly that the idea of loosening his grip terrified him. "I don't know how to do that," he admitted, his voice barely audible.

Amelia squeezed his knees gently before standing up. "Then you need to figure it out, because I can't keep waiting for you to decide whether or not you want to let me in. I care about you, but I need someone who can be all in with me. Not halfway."

Jack looked up at her, the weight of her words settling in his chest like a stone. She wasn't angry—she was hurting, just like he was. And she was right. He had been avoiding his grief, holding on to the pain like it was a lifeline, afraid that letting go would mean starting all over again. That's what depression mean, so afraid of the light that you keep pushing yourself in the more darker places. But in doing so, he was pushing away the people who were still here, still trying to love him.

Amelia grabbed her jacket from the chair and paused at the door, giving him one last, searching look. "I'm not asking for you to have it all figured out, Jack. But you need to at least *try* —for yourself, for us. Otherwise, this isn't going to work."

Jack swallowed hard, the reality of her words sinking in. He nodded, though he wasn't sure what to say. Amelia gave him a small, sad smile before stepping out, leaving him alone in the quiet of his apartment, the echo of their conversation lingering in the empty space.

He sat there for a long time after she left, staring at the floor, the old recording of Liam's band playing faintly in the background. It was like a ghost haunting him, always just out of reach. Jack knew he had to face his fear head-on, but the thought of confronting it felt like staring down a mountain he wasn't sure he could climb. But Amelia was right. If he wanted to move forward—with her, with his life—he needed to start letting go of the fears. And maybe, just maybe, that started by acknowledging that it was okay to live again, despite the bleak hope.

...

The clinking of silverware against plates was the only sound that filled the small, dimly lit kitchen. Jack and Amelia sat across from each other at the table, the half-eaten dinner between them going cold as the silence stretched on. Jack shifted uncomfortably, pushing the food around on his plate, his mind racing but unable to form the right words.

Amelia was the first to speak, her voice soft but carrying an undeniable weight. "Jack, you've been distant again. We've barely talked these last few days." She set her fork down gently, folding her hands in her lap as she studied his face. "What's going on?"

Jack took a deep breath, his chest tightening as he tried to gather his thoughts. He looked down at his plate, feeling the familiar lump of emotion rise in his throat.

"I don't know how to do this," Jack finally said, his voice barely above a whisper. He didn't look up, afraid of what he might see in Amelia's eyes.

Amelia furrowed her brow, leaning in slightly. "Do what?" Jack ran a hand through his hair, exhaling shakily. "I don't know how to love you... fully. I don't know how to be with you without feeling like all of it will crumble again. I'll disappoint you too. Every time I get close to you, it feels like I'm pulling you behind with me. Like I'm choosing to forget you."

Amelia's face softened, but there was a sadness in her eyes. She reached across the table and gently placed her hand on his. "Jack, It's okay to move forward. It doesn't mean you live any less."

Jack shook his head, his eyes still fixed on his plate. "But it feels like…I can't stop thinking about. It's like this fictional memory is always there, between us. I don't know how to love you fully when I'm still so haunted by the past. That you'll start cursing me for doing nothing just like my parents did. You know I've failed everyone in my life. I myself am nothing but a failure. I don't want to ruin your life."

Amelia squeezed his hand, her voice steady but tinged with emotion. "I understand that will always be a part of you. But you're allowed to live your life, Jack. You're allowed to love and live and expect." She paused, searching his face. "But I can't be with you if you're constantly looking over your shoulder, if you're always stuck in the past. I promise I won't fail you. Just always be honest with me. I want nothing but your love. I don't want you to be the man of the house or anything. I know what that's like, I've seen my parents fighting and abusing growing yup"

Jack finally looked up, his eyes glassy with unshed tears. "I don't want to disappoint you, Amelia. You deserve more than what I can give you right now."

Amelia's gaze softened even more, and she gave him a sad smile. "I don't need you to be perfect, Jack. I just need you to try—to let me in. But if you're not ready, then maybe you need time. I don't want to be someone you're just 'trying' with because you feel like you should. I'm asking for the commitment, not essentially a partnership"

The lump in Jack's throat grew tighter, and for a moment, he couldn't breathe. He had known this conversation was coming, but hearing it spoken aloud made the weight of it feel unbearable. He wanted to love Amelia, wanted to move forward, but the past had its claws deep in him, and he didn't know how to let go. "I don't want to lose you," Jack whispered, his voice breaking. "But I don't know how to fix this. You know I'm trying but I can't fix myself completely."

Amelia leaned in, pressing her forehead against his for a moment, closing her eyes. They sat like that for a long moment, the quiet between them filled with unspoken heartache. When Amelia finally pulled away, her eyes were filled with a mixture of love and resignation.

Jack knew this was a crossroads. He could feel it in the air, the weight of the decision pressing down on him. But as much as he wanted to promise her everything, to say he could move past his grief and love her fully, he wasn't sure if he could. Not yet. Amelia stood slowly, her movements deliberate, and kissed him softly on the forehead before walking to the door. "I'll be here when you're ready, Jack," she said quietly. "But don't wait too long."

The door closed softly behind her, leaving Jack alone in the silent kitchen, the remnants of their untouched dinner a painful reminder of what he was on the verge of losing. He sat back in his chair, staring at the door, the ache in his chest growing stronger. For the first time, Jack allowed himself to cry—deep, aching sobs that echoed through the empty room. He didn't know how to move on, but he realized now that if he didn't try, he would lose more than just Amelia. He would lose himself too.

...

One late evening, Sophie and Nate sat together on the porch of Sophie's apartment, the cool breeze brushing against their skin. The day had been long—filled with meetings for the ALS awareness project, shifts at the hospital, and emotional highs and lows—but now, in the stillness of the night, it felt like the world had quieted, leaving just the two of them in this shared moment.

Sophie fiddled with the edge of her sweater, her thoughts swirling in her mind like a storm she couldn't control. Nate sat close beside her, his presence calming, but the weight of her fears still pressed heavy on her chest. She had been holding back for so long—burying her emotions beneath her work, keeping herself too busy to feel too much. But she couldn't keep it buried anymore.

"Nate..." she began, her voice soft, barely above a whisper. She hesitated, her heart racing as she struggled to find the right words. "I... I'm scared."

Nate glanced over at her, his gaze gentle, but he said nothing, waiting for her to continue.

Sophie took a deep breath, her fingers trembling slightly as she spoke. "I'm scared of... of losing people. Of losing you."

Nate's expression softened, and he reached out, his hand finding hers, giving it a comforting squeeze. "Sophie, I'm not going anywhere."

She shook her head, a small, sad smile tugging at the corners of her lips. "I know you say that now, but... I've lost so many people, Nate. First my mom when I was a teen, then Emily. It's like... every time I let someone in, every time I start to care, they get taken away from me. And I don't think I can go through that again."

Her voice cracked on the last word, and she quickly looked down, blinking back the tears that threatened to spill. She hadn't meant to open up like this—it wasn't something she did easily. But with Nate, it felt different. He made her feel safe, like she didn't have to carry the weight of her fears alone.

Nate shifted closer, his thumb gently brushing over her knuckles. "Sophie... I know you've been through a lot. More than anyone should ever have to. And I get why you're scared

—why you want to protect yourself. But you don't have to do it alone." She looked up at him then, her eyes shining with unshed tears. "What if I lose you too?"

He met her gaze, his eyes steady, unwavering. "I can't promise that nothing bad will ever happen. I wish I could. But what I can promise is that I'm here now. And I'm not going to give up on you, Sophie. Not ever. Just like you did, I've fell for you too…way before you did."

The words hit her deeply, a mixture of warmth and fear blooming in her chest. She wanted to believe him—wanted to trust that maybe this time would be different. But the scars of her past, the grief she still carried, made it so hard to let go.

"I don't know if I can do this," she whispered. "I don't know if I can open up and let myself feel everything again."

Nate leaned in closer, his eyes filled with understanding. "We can take things as slow as you need. I'm not in a rush. I just want to be here, with you. Whatever that looks like, however long it takes."

Sophie felt a tear slip down her cheek, and before she could brush it away, Nate reached out, gently wiping it with his thumb. His touch was tender, patient—never pushing her, just offering quiet reassurance. For a long moment, they sat there in silence, the only sound the soft rustling of leaves in the wind. Sophie's heart still felt heavy with the weight of her fears, but for the first time in a long time, there was also a glimmer of hope. Maybe, just maybe, she could let herself try again. Maybe she could trust Nate enough to take that first step. "I'm scared," she repeated, her voice barely audible.

"I know," Nate said softly, leaning his forehead against hers, his breath warm against her skin. "But I'm not. And we'll figure it out together."

Sophie closed her eyes, letting herself rest in the comfort of his words, the steady rhythm of his breathing beside her. For the first time in months, she felt like she didn't have to hold everything together on her own. She didn't have to be perfect, didn't have to be unbreakable. Maybe she could just be. With Nate, maybe that was enough.

Chapter 6: Finding Strength

Jack sat in the sterile, softly lit office, staring at the beige walls and nervously tapping his foot against the floor. This was his second session with Dr. Nguyen, the therapist his doctor had recommended, but it felt like the first real step he had taken toward confronting everything he'd been avoiding. He hadn't wanted to come at first. The idea of talking about his depression, about his fears, about everything he felt but didn't want to feel, had seemed unbearable. But now, sitting across from Dr. Parker, who watched him with patient eyes, Jack knew that he couldn't keep running.

"Where do you want to start today, Jack?" Dr. Nguyen asked gently, her tone non-judgmental, giving him the space to find his words.

Jack swallowed hard, his hands twisting together in his lap. "I don't know," he said after a long pause. "I guess... I guess I still don't know why I'm here. I mean, I know why I'm here. But I don't really know how this is supposed to help."

Dr. Nguyen nodded, her expression calm and encouraging. "That's understandable. Therapy can feel a bit uncomfortable at first, especially when you're dealing with something as deep as depression, bipolar disorder, survivor's guilt. It takes time to work through those feelings."

Jack let out a long, frustrated sigh. "I just keep thinking that it should've been me. Liam... he had so much ahead of him, you know? He had dreams, plans. And now I'm here, trying to live a life that I don't feel like I deserve, while he's... gone…Wait..Am I bipolar? What does that mean"

He paused, his voice catching on the last word, and he quickly blinked away the moisture gathering in his eyes.

"Why do you think it should have been you?" Dr. Nguyen asked, avoiding everything else, her voice soft but probing.

Jack hesitated, running his hands through his hair. "Because he was the better person," he muttered, staring down at the floor. "He was this... larger-than-life guy. He had so much charisma, so much talent. I don't know who I'm supposed to be."

Dr. Nguyen watched him for a moment before responding. "It sounds like you've been carrying the weight of that guilt for a long time, Jack. And it doesn't mean you have to live your life like you owe something to the past."

Jack's jaw clenched. He had heard similar words from Sophie, from Amelia, even from Mason, but they hadn't sunk in.

"But what if I don't know how to move on?" he asked, his voice small and uncertain. "What if I never get past this?"

Dr. Nguyen leaned forward slightly, her gaze steady and compassionate. “Moving on doesn’t mean figuring out everything. Don’t think when you were in depression the world has passed you by. You have the right to live your life, Jack.”

Jack took a shaky breath, the tension in his shoulders easing slightly. “I don’t know how to do that,” he admitted, his voice barely above a whisper.

“It’s not something that happens overnight,” Dr. Nguyen said. “It’s a process. And it starts by letting yourself feel the confidence you’ve been pushing away. You can’t heal what you don’t confront.”

Jack stared at the floor, his chest tight with the weight of her words. He had spent so long avoiding this—distracting himself with work, relationships, anything that kept him from facing the depth of his fears and darkness. But now, sitting here, he realized that maybe it was time to stop running.

“I want to try,” he said quietly, almost to himself. “I don’t know if I’m ready, but... I want to try.”

Dr. Nguyen gave him a small, encouraging smile. “That’s a good place to start, Jack. We’ll take it one step at a time.” Jack nodded, the knots of guilt and grief still tangled inside him, but for the first time, he felt a flicker of hope. Maybe he didn’t have to carry this burden alone anymore. Maybe he could finally start healing. He could be the better person.

...

Sophie’s decision to take a leave of absence from her relentless activism work was both difficult and liberating. For years, she had thrown herself into every project, every cause, all in the name of honouring Emily's memory and help those diagnosed with the disease, but it had left her exhausted, mentally and emotionally drained. Taking a step back was like exhaling after holding her breath for far too long. With Nate by her side, she finally began to explore life outside of the hospitals and awareness campaigns. Their relationship, once filled with hesitation and Sophie's fear of losing him, started to deepen naturally, evolving from partnership into something more solid and fulfilling. Nate was patient, letting Sophie set the pace, but he also encouraged her to find joy in the little things again.

They began to take on small adventures together, beginning with hiking, something Sophie had never considered before. Their first hike was a local trail, the kind of easy, scenic path lined with tall trees and soft breezes. Sophie felt out of place at first, awkward in her hiking boots, feeling guilty about enjoying herself. But Nate was there, cracking jokes as they stumbled over rocks and tree roots, making the whole experience lighthearted. He teased her when she couldn't figure out the compass on her phone, and they laughed when they realized they'd been walking in circles for twenty minutes. For the first time in what felt like forever, Sophie smiled, a genuine, carefree smile that surprised even her.

As they grew more comfortable in each other's presence, they started cooking together—though cooking might've been a generous term for what was actually happening. Their kitchen adventures were filled with burnt pots and over-salted dishes, Nate fumbling with the instructions while Sophie pretended to be the master chef. One night, they attempted a complicated pasta recipe that quickly turned into a hilarious disaster. Flour covered the counters, the sauce boiled over, and at one point, the fire alarm went off as their garlic bread charred to a crisp. Nate, in his usual calm way, shrugged it off, tossing the burnt bread in the trash and suggesting they order takeout instead. Sophie couldn't stop laughing, her stomach aching as they collapsed on the couch with pizza boxes, feeling like they had won some small, silly victory.

Their travels followed, small weekend trips to nearby towns, exploring places Sophie had never seen before. They visited quiet, tucked-away bed-and-breakfasts, took long drives along the coast, and found themselves wandering through local markets and hidden cafes. There was something peaceful about being away from the intensity of her previous life, something refreshing about seeing the world through a lens that wasn't tinted with grief or responsibility. Nate's presence during all of this wasn't overwhelming. He never pushed her too far but instead allowed her to rediscover joy at her own pace. Whether they were hiking up a mountain, attempting to bake a cake, or sitting by the ocean watching the sunset, Sophie felt herself letting go bit by bit, learning to embrace happiness without the constant weight of loss pulling her back.

She still had her moments—times when the memories of the guilt, and the anxiety would creep back into her mind. But now, instead of pushing those feelings away or burying them beneath work, Sophie had Nate. And more importantly, she had herself, a version of herself she was just starting to get to know again. The more they spent time together, the more Sophie realized that it was okay to lean on someone else, to let herself love and be loved without the fear of losing it all. Her relationship with Nate wasn't about forgetting Emily or her activism; it was about finding balance—about remembering that it was okay to live, to feel joy, and to move forward without letting go of the past completely.

Sophie and Nate's road trip started off like any other, with good intentions and a carefully planned route. But somewhere between trying to find the perfect scenic overlook and stopping for gas in the middle of nowhere, things went hilariously off track. What was supposed to be a quick two-hour drive to a quaint coastal town turned into a comedy of errors, starting with Sophie's insistence on "taking the scenic route" and Nate's less-than-ideal navigation skills.

It began when they missed a crucial turn and wound up on a winding back road, lined with fields that seemed to stretch forever. The GPS was no help, recalculating their route every few miles with an unhelpful robotic voice that Sophie swore was getting sassier by the minute. Nate, trying to play it cool, assured Sophie that they weren't lost—they were just "exploring new territory."

After nearly an hour of "exploring," they pulled into a tiny, one-stoplight town. The place looked like something out of a Hallmark movie—charming in an oddly over-the-top way, complete with a small-town diner, a general store, and the most eccentric bed-and-breakfast they'd ever seen. The B&B was an old, Victorian-style house painted in bright pastel colours, with a sign out front that read *"Welcome to Petunia Place: A Home for Strays (and Tourists)"*.

Laughing at the ridiculousness of the situation, they decided to check in for the night. The owner, Mrs. Petunia herself, was an elderly woman with a penchant for knitting and a collection of bizarre cat-themed decor that filled every corner of the house. There were cat pillows, cat clocks, even cat-shaped salt and pepper shakers on the dining room table.

Sophie could barely hold back her laughter as Mrs. Petunia showed them to their room—decorated, of course, with even more cat memorabilia.

That night, they found themselves in the quirkiest of situations. The B&B hosted "Storytime by the Fire," where Mrs. Petunia gathered her guests (all three of them) to share local folklore and tales of the town's history. Nate, ever the good sport, tried his best to look interested as Mrs. Petunia enthusiastically described the legend of *"Catspaw Hill,"* a supposedly haunted hill just outside town where a family of cats once "saved" the village from an unexplained disaster. Sophie, on the other hand, had to fake a coughing fit to cover her giggles.

The next morning, over a breakfast of oddly shaped pancakes (cat-shaped, naturally), Sophie and Nate reflected on their accidental detour. While it hadn't been the romantic, picturesque getaway they'd planned, it was one of the most fun and memorable experiences they'd shared. Getting lost had led them to Petunia Place—a place they would never have chosen on purpose but one they were now glad to have stumbled upon.

As they got back on the road, Sophie joked that maybe they should let Nate navigate more often if it meant finding more weird and wonderful places like Petunia Place. Nate, with his classic deadpan humour, replied, "Only if you're okay with more haunted hills and cat pancakes." They laughed, the kind of laughter that came easily now, filled with warmth and lightness. It was moments like these that reminded Sophie of why she had fallen for Nate—the ability to find joy, even when things went hilariously off course.

...

One quiet evening, Jack and Amelia sat together in his small apartment, the soft glow of string lights casting a warm hue across the room. The city outside buzzed with life, but inside, everything felt still and intimate. Jack hadn't been distant lately, caught in his usual battle with the ghosts of his past, and tonight felt different. He was tired of avoiding the inevitable conversation that had been building between them for months.

As they sat on the couch, Jack turned to Amelia, his eyes filled with a mix of hesitation and hope. "I've been holding onto so much for so long," he began, his voice quiet but steady. "Everything that happened... it's always felt like this huge weight I couldn't get past. Like if I moved on, I'd be again ending up in the bad place somehow."

Amelia, ever patient, listened carefully, sensing that this was the moment Jack had been building up to. But she had also seen the good in him—the kind, thoughtful man who, beneath the layers of grief and guilt, had so much love to give.

"You're being enough, Jack" she said softly. "You're allowed to live. You're allowed to be happy."

Jack nodded, a small smile breaking through as he spoke, "I think I'm finally starting to realize that. I've been holding myself back, stuck in this place where I'm scared to move forward because I thought it would mean letting go. But now I wouldn't want that for me either? You know our brain is made of uncountable parts, like car you can fix easily but brain? There's no guarantee."

Jack reached for her hand, the weight of his confession lifting slowly from his shoulders. "I'm ready to start living again. For us."

Amelia squeezed his hand, her heart swelling with relief and joy. It had taken so long to get to this point, but hearing Jack say those words felt like the breakthrough they both needed. For so long, their relationship had been marked by caution and hesitation, by the ghosts of the past. But now, it felt like they were finally stepping into something real, something full of promise.

As they sat there, hands intertwined, the silence between them was filled with a sense of peace. Jack wasn't running anymore—he was facing his grief head-on and choosing to move forward. And in doing so, he was choosing Amelia.

Their relationship blossomed in the weeks that followed, no longer weighed down by the past. It wasn't perfect—there were still moments when Jack would get quiet, when memories of his depression days resurfaced—but they were growing, together. Their connection deepened, built on a foundation of honesty and mutual understanding. Jack found himself smiling more, laughing more, feeling lighter than he had in years. And Amelia, who had stood by him through his darkest days, was there for it all, her steady presence a source of strength.

They shared quiet mornings over coffee, late-night talks filled with dreams for the future, and moments of simple joy —like cooking dinner together or walking hand in hand through the park. It was steady, it was beautiful, and for the first time in a long time, Jack felt like he was truly living again. Amelia brought him back to life, and Jack, in turn, was ready to love her fully. This was the beginning of something real, something they both knew could last.

Chapter 7: Moving Forward

When Sophie returned to the hospital upon Alysaa's call that she missed her and wanted to meet, her mind was heavy with the memories of Emily, but she was determined to do better this time. She walked into the sterile hallways, where the sound of beeping monitors and hushed voices filled the air. Her first stop was Alyssa's room, a young woman in her early twenties who had been diagnosed with early-stage COPD, but whose condition had taken a turn for the worse in last few days.

Alyssa had become more than just a patient to Sophie; she was a reminder of the life Sophie had fought to save with Emily. The resemblance in their fighting spirits was uncanny. Despite the setbacks, Alyssa's positivity and resilience shone through. She had a bright smile that never seemed to dim, even as her breath came in short, laboured gasps.

Today, Alyssa was scheduled for a new round of treatments. Sophie watched as the respiratory team prepped the nebulizer for her breathing treatment. She monitored Alyssa's vitals closely, paying special attention to her oxygen saturation levels, making notes in her chart. The numbers weren't promising, and Sophie felt her chest tighten. She adjusted the mask over Alyssa's face, offering words of encouragement.

"You're stronger than you think, Alyssa. We'll get through this," Sophie said, her voice soft but firm.

Alyssa's eyes met Sophie's, the fear in them evident. "It's getting harder to breathe, Sophie," she admitted between shallow breaths. "I don't want to die."

Sophie's heart ached. The fear in Alyssa's voice mirrored what she had heard from Emily during those final days. But this time, Sophie wouldn't crumble. She pulled a chair up beside Alyssa's bed, gripping her hand tightly. "You're not alone. I'm with you, every step of the way." As the hours passed, Alyssa's condition worsened. The doctors had prescribed corticosteroids to help with inflammation, and Sophie had made sure the dosage was correct. The medication was strong, intended to ease Alyssa's breathing, but Sophie knew from experience that there were limits. She reviewed the prescriptions again—long-acting bronchodilators, corticosteroids, oxygen therapy—but despite their best efforts, Alyssa's oxygen levels continued to drop. Sophie felt the familiar helplessness creeping in, the same feeling she had experienced with Emily.

Dr. Liam Harp, the specialist Sophie had consulted in the past, was called in to oversee the case. As he reviewed Alyssa's chart, he gave Sophie a sympathetic glance. "We're doing everything we can, but the progression is faster than we anticipated," he explained. "This is the tough part—waiting to see how she responds." Sophie stayed beside Alyssa as the hours turned into a gruelling night. She reassured her, checked the machines, and adjusted her oxygen levels when needed. Alyssa's condition reached a critical point during the night. Her breath was shallow, her skin pale, and Sophie could feel the weight of the moment pressing down on her.

"Alyssa, we're increasing your oxygen," Sophie said, gently adjusting the oxygen mask, trying to keep her voice steady.

Alyssa nodded weakly. "Thank you," she whispered. Sophie updated Dr. Harp on the situation, discussing the next steps and possible changes in medication. But the truth was hard to face—there was only so much that could be done. The doctors recommended increasing Alyssa's dosage of bronchodilators and introducing mechanical ventilation, a step Sophie knew would be a last resort.

Late in the night, Sophie sat by Alyssa's side, refusing to leave her. Memories of Emily's unfilled prescriptions, hidden away in her hospital bag, flooded her mind. The guilt she carried felt like a heavy burden, but this time she was determined not to fail. She leaned in close to Alyssa, wiping a tear from the young woman's cheek. "I'm here. I'm not going anywhere, I'll take care of you myself. It's alright to feel hopeless and bad with all the medications" she whispered.

As the night wore on, Sophie saw the toll the disease was taking. Her heart ached, but she remained strong for Alyssa. In the hardest moments, Sophie realized that, while she couldn't change the outcome, being there was what truly mattered—offering comfort, strength, and hope even when hope felt distant. Dr. Harp reassured Sophie that they were doing everything medically possible, but as the sun rose, Sophie knew the fight wasn't over. She stayed by Alyssa's side, offering comfort through every breathless moment, refusing to let go.

...

Jack's bond with Noah deepened as they spent more time together. The boy, once so withdrawn and resistant to the ways of therapy, had slowly begun to open up. Their sessions had transformed from tense silences into meaningful conversations, and music had played a pivotal role in breaking down those barriers. Jack had always believed in the power of music—it had been his escape during his darkest times, and now, it was Noah's.

One afternoon, after another breakthrough session where Noah shared memories of his parents for the first time, Jack had an idea. He proposed incorporating music therapy into their work, not just for Noah, but for the other kids at the centre. It was something he'd been thinking about for a while, a way to honour memories without being trapped by it.

Music had been Liam's passion, and Jack still remembered the way his friend would lose himself in a song, strumming his guitar late into the night. Liam's band had been a major part of his life, and Jack realized that music could be just as therapeutic for others as it had been for them.

Jack decided to pitch the idea to Mason, who had become his closest confidant at the youth centre. Together, they worked on designing a program that would use music therapy as a tool for emotional expression and healing. They gathered a collection of instruments—guitars, keyboards, drums—and began incorporating music into their group sessions.

Noah, in particular, took to the music therapy. His reluctance slowly melted away as he learned to play simple melodies, and Jack watched with pride as the boy's confidence grew. Their bond had become something more than just therapist and patient—it was a relationship built on trust, shared loss, and the healing power of music. For Jack, the project became more than just a professional endeavour. It was personal. Music had always been the one thing that helped him cope with his own emotions, and now, he was using it to help others do the same. In a way, he felt like he was keeping Liam's legacy alive, but instead of being haunted by the memory, he found peace in it. The music therapy program quickly gained momentum at the centre, with more kids joining in each week. Jack began incorporating songwriting into their sessions, encouraging the teens to put their emotions into lyrics. Some wrote about their grief, others about their hopes, and a few even found humour in the process. Jack saw how music was giving them an outlet for their pain, and it was deeply rewarding.

As Jack sat with the kids, strumming guitar and guiding them through songs, he felt something shift within him. The weight of depression that had once felt unbearable had begun to lift. Liam's memory was still there, but it no longer felt like a burden. Instead, it was a source of comfort, a reminder of the love and friendship that would always be a part of him. For the first time in a long time, Jack felt a sense of purpose. Through music, he was helping these kids navigate their own anxieties, just as he had learned to navigate his own. And as he watched Noah smile while playing a simple tune, Jack knew that he was finally finding peace— with his own life moving forward.

…

One evening, after another long day of working on ALS and COPD projects, Sophie and Nate found themselves sitting on the porch of Sophie's apartment. The night air was cool and quiet, and the stars shimmered faintly above them. It had been a busy few months, but there was a calm between them, a kind of peace that Sophie hadn't felt in a long time.

Nate leaned back in his chair, glancing over at Sophie, who seemed lost in thought. "You've been quieter than usual tonight," he said softly. "Everything okay?"

Sophie turned to him, her eyes reflecting the gentle glow of the porch light. She felt the familiar stir of fear in her chest, the same fear that had kept her from fully opening up to Nate, even after everything they'd shared. She had spent so long holding back, afraid of letting herself get too close, too vulnerable. Nate had been patient with her, never pushing, always giving her the space to breathe. He made her laugh when she needed it most, and he had become her rock when the waves of grief threatened to pull her under. Slowly, steadily, he had shown her that she didn't have to carry the burden of her past alone.

Sophie took a deep breath, her heart pounding as she searched for the right words. She looked into Nate's eyes, and for the first time in a long time, she didn't feel the overwhelming fear of losing someone she cared about. Instead, she felt...hope.

"Nate," she began, her voice soft but steady, "I've been scared for a long time. Scared to let myself feel anything real because... because I didn't want to lose again. But I'm starting to realize that holding back hasn't protected me from the pain —it's only kept me from living. I love you. I want to have a family"

Nate listened quietly, his eyes never leaving hers. He didn't say anything, but the warmth in his gaze gave her the courage to keep going.

"I've been so focused on trying to stay strong, on not letting anyone in because I thought it would hurt too much if I did. But the truth is... I'm tired of being afraid. I'm tired of pushing away the people who care about me."

Her voice wavered for a moment, but she pressed on, determined to be honest—for herself and for him.

"I don't know what the future holds, and I can't promise that I won't be scared sometimes. But I do know that I want to let myself love again. And I want to love you, Nate."

There. She'd said it. The words she'd been holding back for so long, the words she was terrified to admit. But as they hung in the air between them, Sophie didn't feel fear. Instead, she felt a sense of relief, as if a weight had been lifted from her shoulders. Nate's face softened, and a slow, gentle smile spread across his lips. He reached over and took her hand in his, his touch warm and steady. "Sophie, I've been waiting for you to say that, but I never wanted to rush you. I know how hard this has been for you. But I'm here. I've always been here, and I'm not going anywhere."

Sophie smiled through the tears that had begun to well up in her eyes. For the first time in what felt like forever, she allowed herself to fully feel the warmth of Nate's presence, to let him in completely. As they sat there together, hand in hand, under the vast expanse of stars, Sophie knew she was finally ready to take the risk, to open her heart and let love back in. It wasn't about forgetting the pain of the past, but about choosing to live despite it—about embracing the love she still had to give, without fear of what might come next.

Chapter 8: Healing

Jack and Amelia stood at the edge of the beach, the sound of the waves gently lapping against the shore. It was quiet, save for the rhythmic hum of the ocean, a place of solace where Jack had spent so many summers in childhood. Jack had been hesitant about returning, but Amelia had suggested the trip, sensing it was something he needed, even if he didn't realize it himself.

The sun was just beginning to set, casting golden hues across the sky. Jack took a deep breath, his hands in his pockets as he gazed out at the horizon. For the first time, the beach didn't feel like a place haunted by memories. Instead, it felt peaceful, not in a way that weighed Jack down, but in a way that reminded him of the beauty of life and living.

Amelia walked over to him, her hand gently slipping into his. She didn't say anything, allowing him the space to process. They'd been together for months now, but Jack still felt as if a part of him had been holding back, too tangled up in his depression to fully be present. Amelia, patient and understanding, had given him time—more than anyone else might have. But this trip was different. Jack could feel something shifting inside of him.

They wandered down the beach together, the soft sand beneath their feet as they walked in comfortable silence. Jack glanced over at Amelia, her hair tousled by the breeze, her expression calm but knowing. She had a way of being there without pushing, a quiet strength that he admired.

After a while, they found a spot to sit, overlooking the ocean as the last light of the day faded into twilight. Jack pulled out a small notebook from his jacket pocket, something he'd been carrying with him since they'd arrived. It was filled with old notes for future from his childhood—diary of sorts but written inconsistently and momentarily. Jack had held onto it, never quite ready to look through it, but now, it felt like the right time.

He opened it, running his fingers over the pages, the scribbled handwriting bringing a flood of memories. As he read through some notes, some unfinished, some complete, he felt a warmth spread through him. These weren't just reminders of his past—they were pieces of his lost life. His creativity, his laughter, his love for living.

Amelia watched him quietly, sensing the importance of the moment. After a while, Jack spoke, his voice soft but steady. "I used to think that holding onto this stuff, holding onto the past, was the only way to keep dreams with me. But I think... maybe it's time to let go of the guilt that I didn't make the most of it." Amelia leaned in closer, her shoulder brushing his. "Letting go doesn't mean forgetting, Jack. It means honouring memory by being here." Jack nodded, the weight in his chest finally starting to lift. "I think I'm finally ready to start living again. Start anew."

As they sat there, the sound of the waves filling the quiet between them, Jack realized he wasn't alone in this journey. Amelia had been his anchor, steady and unwavering, helping him find his way back to himself. Their bond had grown deeper with every passing day, but it was in this moment, on this beach that he had loved life so much, that Jack felt like he could finally be fully present with her. He turned to Amelia, his eyes softening. "I don't know where this is going, but I know that I want you with me. All of this... it feels different now. Like I can finally breathe again." Amelia smiled, her hand resting over his. "We'll figure it out together. There's no rush. Just... be here now."

Jack nodded, feeling more at peace than he had in years. The grief of depression would always be there, a part of him, but it no longer defined him. For the first time, he felt like he could carry his life forward, without being trapped by the past for that nothing went as he had planned out, there just wasn't that spirit. As the night descended, Jack leaned back, his hand still intertwined with Amelia's, the ocean stretching out before them, endless and full of possibilities.

...

At the ALS conference, the auditorium was packed with doctors, researchers, patients, and advocates, all gathered to hear about the latest advancements and share their experiences. The air buzzed with a mix of excitement and solemnity—an understanding that, while progress had been made, there was still much to be done in the fight against ALS. Sophie stood backstage, her heart racing.

The emcee introduced her, and as Sophie stepped onto the stage, the room fell silent. The lights were bright, but she could still see faces looking back at her—some familiar, some not. She took a deep breath, gripping the edges of the podium for support, her notes lying untouched beside her. For a moment, the weight of everything—her journey, her grief, her activism—pressed down on her. But then she thought of Liam's easy smile, Emily's infectious laugh, and how far she had come since their loss.

"I never thought I'd be here," she began, her voice strong but soft. "I never thought I'd be the one standing in front of all of you, telling my story. But here I am, not just for myself, but for the people who couldn't be here—for Liam, and for Emily, and for the patients I got to care for."

She paused, scanning the crowd, feeling the emotions well up inside her but refusing to let them overwhelm her. "Liam was... someone you couldn't forget. He was my best friend and an incredible musician, full of dreams. Emily, on the other hand, was like a sister to me—strong, funny, a fighter until the end. Both of them faced ALS and COPD with courage I can't begin to describe, but what I want to share with you today isn't just about their struggle. It's about what they taught me."

Sophie shared stories of late-night hospital visits, the way Liam never let ALS steal his love for music, and how Emily, even when her breath became too shallow to speak, still managed to crack jokes. She talked about the hardest moments—finding Emily's hidden, unfilled prescriptions, the helplessness she felt as a nurse watching her friends suffer, knowing there were limits to what she could do.

"But despite everything, Liam and Emily didn't let their illnesses define them," Sophie said, her voice shaking slightly as she fought back tears. "They lived fully, even in the hardest moments, and that's why I'm here. To make sure that their stories live on through this work, through the awareness we raise, and the research we support."

The room was silent, every eye on her. She could feel the shared understanding in the crowd, the empathy that connected them all. Sophie knew that many of the people in the audience had their own stories of loss, of hope, of resilience.

"As someone who's been in both positions—a caregiver and a friend—I know the toll these diseases take, not just physically, but emotionally. But what I've learned is that the only way we truly lose someone is if we forget them. So I'm here to honour Liam and Emily and Alyssa and my patients by making sure no one else forgets them."

Sophie glanced down at the small bracelet on her wrist, one she had made in memory of Alyssa. She had given the same bracelet to Nate before the conference, a small gesture that symbolized how far she had come—not just in her work, but in allowing herself to heal and grow closer to those she loved.

"I know now that Liam and Emily wouldn't want me to be stuck in grief. They would want me to live, to keep fighting, and to help others do the same. And that's what I'll continue to do."

As she finished, the room erupted in applause, but for Sophie, it was more than just a reaction to her words. It felt like closure, like she was finally at peace with the path she had chosen. Walking off the stage, she felt lighter, knowing that she was honouring both Alyssa and Emily—not by holding onto the pain, but by turning it into something that could help others. Nate was waiting for her backstage, a quiet smile on his face. "You were incredible," he whispered, pulling her into a gentle embrace. Sophie nodded, feeling the weight of the moment lift from her shoulders. She felt at peace, knowing that she was exactly where she was meant to be.

...

The reunion took place on a cloudy afternoon in the youth center's modest courtyard, the air heavy with anticipation. Jack stood beside Noah, his heart pounding in sync with the boy's. Noah, normally so guarded, looked nervous—his small hands fidgeting in his pockets, his face a mix of hope and fear. Jack had never seen him like this. Over the past few months, their bond had deepened, but this was something new, something more vulnerable. Noah's mother, Claire, arrived with hesitation in her step, her eyes scanning the area until they landed on Noah. Her face softened, the years of estrangement melting away in a single glance. She hadn't seen him since he was a little boy, and now here he was—older, more closed off, but still her son.

Jack gave Noah a reassuring nod. "She's here for you, buddy," he said softly, stepping back to give them space.

Noah swallowed hard, his eyes darting from Jack to Claire. He was scared, Jack could tell. Scared of being rejected again, of hoping too much. But there was also a glimmer of something else—something fragile, like a seed of hope ready to take root.

Claire knelt down to Noah's level, her voice trembling as she spoke. "Noah, I've missed you so much."

Noah blinked, his expression unreadable. "Why didn't you come sooner?" His voice was small, filled with the pain of years spent feeling forgotten.

Claire's eyes filled with tears, her hand reaching out but stopping just short of touching him, as if she was afraid she didn't have the right. "I wanted to, Noah. I did. But I didn't know how. After your father…" She paused, swallowing back the lump in her throat. "I was scared. I didn't know if you'd even want me in your life after everything. But I'm here now, and if you'll let me, I want to be there for you."

The silence between them stretched, heavy with emotion. Jack held his breath, watching, hoping.

Noah's face crumpled. "I thought you didn't care about me anymore."

Claire's hand finally closed the gap, resting gently on Noah's shoulder. "I've always cared, Noah. I'm so sorry I didn't show it sooner. But I'm here now, and I'm not going anywhere."

Tears welled up in Noah's eyes, and for the first time since Jack had met him, he let them fall. Claire wrapped her arms around him, pulling him into a hug that felt long overdue.

Noah hesitated for a moment, but then he buried his face in her shoulder, clinging to her as if afraid she might disappear again. Jack felt his own throat tighten as he watched the scene unfold. It was a moment of hope—hope for Noah, for Claire, and for a future where the boy didn't have to feel so alone anymore.

As they held each other, the clouds overhead began to part, letting the rays of sunlight filter through. Jack smiled to himself, feeling a warmth spread through his chest. For so long, Noah had kept his heart locked away, refusing to let anyone in. But now, with Claire, it seemed like he finally had a chance at something stable, something loving.

After a while, Claire stood, keeping her arm around Noah's shoulders. She looked over at Jack, her expression filled with gratitude. "Thank you," she mouthed silently. Jack nodded, his heart full. He had given Noah a chance at something better—something every kid deserved: a family, a home, and the hope of brighter days ahead.

Chapter 9: Home

Sophie and Jack stood side by side in the peaceful cemetery, the autumn air cool and crisp. The trees surrounding them had started to change colours, shades of orange and gold painting the landscape. It had been a long time since they'd visited Liam and Emily's graves together, and even though the pain still lingered, it felt different now. Softer, less raw.

Sophie gently placed a bouquet of white lilies at Emily's headstone, her fingers tracing the engraved name, and smiled softly, her eyes filled with a mixture of love and loss. "Emily would laugh if she saw how many times I've messed up trying to cook lately," Sophie said, her voice light with humour but tinged with a lingering sadness. "She was always the one who made sure I didn't burn everything."

Jack chuckled beside her, his hands shoved into his jacket pockets as he stood in front of Liam's grave. "Liam used to say that cooking was just like playing music—both take rhythm. But I think he forgot I was the one who always had two left feet." He smiled, looking down at the stone, a warmth spreading through him as he remembered all their shared moments. "You know, I started bringing guitar to the youth centre. Teaching the kids a bit of what he taught me. I think he'd get a kick out of that."

Sophie's smile grew. "He'd love that." She glanced at Jack, noticing the calm in his eyes that wasn't there the last time they'd come here. "You're doing good, Jack. I'm proud of you."

Jack nodded, feeling a warmth in his chest. "I'm proud of you too, Sophie. Emily would be so proud of all the work you've done, the lives you've helped." He paused, taking a breath. "I know you've been through hell, but… you've come out the other side. We both have."

Sophie swallowed, her throat tightening as tears welled up in her eyes. "I still miss her every day," she admitted, her voice trembling slightly. "There are times when it feels like no matter what I do, it's never enough to fill the space she left behind."

Jack's expression softened. "I know what you mean. There are still nights when I dream about Liam, and for a second, I wake up thinking he's still here." He let out a slow breath, looking up at the sky. "But we're here, Soph. We're still standing. And we're living and that in a way honours them."

They stood in silence for a moment, the weight of their grief mixing with the quiet peace of knowing they'd found their way through it and complexities of their own life. Sophie tucked a strand of hair behind her ear, her hand resting lightly on Emily's headstone.

"I think we've come a long way," she said softly. "It hasn't been easy, but... we're finally learning how to live again."

Jack nodded in agreement. "And that's all they would have wanted for us."

Sophie's gaze drifted across the cemetery, her heart heavy but steady. "I'm glad we've stayed friends," she said, a small smile tugging at her lips. "After everything, it's good to know we're still here for each other."

"Always," Jack replied, his voice filled with sincerity. "We've been through too much to lose that."

As the wind rustled the leaves around them, they both felt a sense of closure, not in forgetting, but in carrying forward the love and memories of Liam and Emily. They had both found new paths, new people to love, but what they shared with their lost friends would always be a part of them, something that has shaped their life. And for the first time in a long while, they didn't feel guilty about it. They felt at peace.

...

Jack and Amelia sat on the porch of her small apartment, the sun beginning to set over the horizon, casting a warm golden glow across the city. The evening air was cool, and the sound of distant traffic filled the silence between them. Jack turned to Amelia, his hands resting on the armrests of his chair, feeling the weight of the conversation they'd been skirting around for weeks now.

Amelia glanced over at him, her eyes soft but curious. She could sense something was on his mind. "You've been quiet today," she said gently, her fingers brushing a stray lock of hair behind her ear. "What's going on?"

Jack shifted in his seat, his heart racing a little, but this time it wasn't out of fear or uncertainty. He had finally come to a place where the idea of moving forward didn't feel like a burden. It felt like living, like finally breathing again.

"I've been thinking," he began, his voice steady but low. "About us. About our future." He paused, meeting her gaze, seeing the flicker of anticipation in her eyes. "I know things have been complicated, with everything that's happened, but... I'm ready, Amelia. I'm ready to start building something real. With you."

Amelia's eyes softened, her expression a mix of surprise and warmth. "Jack... are you sure? I know how hard it's been for you, and I don't want to rush anything." Jack nodded, his hand reaching out to take hers, their fingers intertwining. "I've thought about it a lot. I've been not living for so long, but that depression is not weighing me down anymore. It's still there, it always will be or not, but... I'm ready to live again. To try. To live fully." He paused, looking into her eyes with all the honesty he could muster. "And I want to live that life with you."

Amelia squeezed his hand, her lips curving into a soft, loving smile. "I've wanted this for so long, but I didn't want to push. I wanted you to come to it on your own."

"I know," Jack replied, his voice filled with gratitude. "You've been patient, more than I deserved sometimes. But I'm here now, and I'm not holding back anymore. I want us to move in together, to start building a home. I want to make plans, talk about our future—where we're going, what we want. I'm ready for all of it."

Amelia's eyes glistened as she blinked back tears. "I want that too, Jack. I've always wanted that with you." For the first time in what felt like forever, Jack felt a deep sense of calm and excitement wash over him. The weight of the past had lifted, and in its place, a future with Amelia began to take shape. They had both waited so long, and now, the path ahead didn't feel so uncertain anymore. It felt full of possibility.

"I love you," Jack said, his voice firm and filled with conviction. "I want us to build something beautiful together."

Amelia leaned in, kissing him softly. "I love you too," she whispered against his lips. "Let's do this." And just like that, their future began to unfold. Together.

Chapter 10: Finding Where We Belong

The soft hues of early morning light filtered through the windows as Sophie and Jack both stood at pivotal crossroads in their lives. The gentle warmth of a new day mirrored the quiet peace that had finally settled over them—each in their own way, after years of navigating grief, uncertainty, and personal battles.

Sophie stood in the small living room of Nate's apartment, her hands nervously gripping a tiny box wrapped in a simple ribbon. She had thought about this moment for days, wondering how she would feel, what she would say. The air was thick with a blend of excitement and apprehension, but today, she felt ready. Ready to take a step forward, not just in her relationship with Nate, but in her healing journey.

Nate was in the kitchen, humming a tune to himself as he brewed coffee. He had no idea what Sophie had planned, no clue that this seemingly ordinary afternoon would carry such meaning. She had grown to cherish these quiet moments with him, the simple routines they'd begun to share as they got closer. But today, she wanted to give him something that showed her deeper commitment—a small, meaningful gesture to acknowledge their love, but also everything that had brought them to this point.

"Hey," Sophie called, her voice a little shaky but warm, "Can you come here for a second?"

Nate turned, wiping his hands on a dish towel as he approached her, a curious smile on his face. "What's up?" he asked, noticing the slight tremble in her hands and the small box she held. Sophie took a deep breath, her heart racing in anticipation. She hadn't expected to feel so emotional about this moment, but as she looked at him, she realized how far they had come—how far she had come. "I've been thinking a lot," she started, her voice soft but steady. "About us. About... everything. And I wanted to give you something."

Nate's eyes softened, the curiosity in his gaze now mixed with something more tender. "Sophie... you didn't have to get me anything."

"I know," she said, smiling nervously as she handed him the small box. "But I wanted to. It's something that means a lot to me, and I hope it'll mean something to you too."

Nate carefully untied the ribbon, opening the box to reveal a small, delicate pendant. It wasn't flashy or overly ornate, just a simple silver charm shaped like a heart intertwined with an infinity symbol. With a note that he's going to be a father. On the back, there was a small engraving: *Love. Strength. Resilience.*

Later that evening, Jack and Amelia sat on the beach, watching the sun dip below the horizon. The sound of the waves was calming, and Jack felt at peace. He had made the decision to move in with Amelia, a choice that once terrified him but now felt right. She had been patient, understanding of his fears, but more importantly, she had helped him see that it was okay to live fully, even after loss.

Amelia leaned her head on his shoulder, her voice soft as she spoke. "You've come a long way, Jack. Most people don't." Jack smiled, his heart swelling with gratitude and love. "And I think I'm finally ready for whatever comes next."

On the other side of town, Sophie and Nate sat on their porch, enjoying the quiet of the evening. Sophie glanced at Nate, a content smile on her face. "I never thought I'd get here," she admitted quietly, her fingers brushing the pendant she now wore around her neck. "But I finally feel like I belong."

Nate smiled, wrapping an arm around her. "You've always belonged, Sophie. You just had to find your way back." As the stars began to twinkle in the night sky, both Sophie and Jack felt a deep sense of peace. They had found where they belonged—not just in their careers, but in the love and connections they had rebuilt. Their lives, though scarred by loss, were now filled with hope and purpose. And as they looked toward the future, they knew they were ready to face it with open hearts, carrying the memories of Liam and Emily with them, not as burdens, but as beacons guiding them forward.

…

In a cozy, dimly lit restaurant. The small, round table is scattered with half-empty plates, a few glasses of wine, and the sound of easy, carefree laughter filling the air. Sophie, Nate, Jack, and Amelia sit together, their faces glowing with the warmth of shared memories and the joy of having each other.

Sophie leans back in her chair, her eyes sparkling as she recounts the latest misadventure she and Nate experienced on their road trip. "So, we're driving through this tiny town, right? And Nate insists we don't need a map or GPS—'I've got a sense of direction like a hawk,' he says." She shoots Nate a teasing grin, who, in mock defensiveness, crosses his arms.

"Hey, I stand by that," Nate retorts with a playful smirk. "It was just a minor detour."

"A minor detour?" Sophie laughs, leaning toward Amelia. "We ended up at some ancient bed-and-breakfast run by this woman who swore the place was haunted! I was convinced the walls were going to start talking."

Jack, who had been listening with a grin, chimes in. "Wait, wait—haunted? You didn't hear anything spooky, did you?"

Nate shakes his head, chuckling. "No ghosts, but the bed was so squeaky I thought it was going to collapse every time we moved. It was like being in a 1920s horror flick."

Amelia giggles, shaking her head. "Oh my God, Nate! You could've at least listened to Sophie about using a map. It's 2036—who even navigates by instinct anymore?"

Sophie leans in, trying to suppress her laughter. "It was the squeak. I swear, I barely slept. Every time Nate turned over, it was like—" She makes a loud creaking noise, mimicking the bed, and they all burst out laughing.

Jack, wiping tears of laughter from his eyes, adds, "Well, at least it wasn't a reunion with Mason's terrible jokes."

"Oh God, please no," Spphie groans, dramatically rolling his eyes. "I don't think I could handle another one of those awful puns about guitars."

"Remember when he tried to work one of those jokes into his speech at the youth centre?" Sophie says, her shoulders shaking with laughter. "He was so serious, too. Everyone was trying to be polite, but it was just so bad."

Nate looks at Jack, who raises his glass with a grin. "To squeaky beds, haunted B&Bs, and Mason's legendary puns," he says, and the group toasts with their glasses, clinking together in a moment that feels almost surreal. There's no heaviness in the air, no lingering pain from the past. Just the four of them friends —two couples, laughing and joking like they hadn't in years.

Sophie catches Nate's eye and smiles, feeling lighter than she ever imagined she could. Jack, meanwhile, squeezes Amelia's hand under the table, knowing that he, too, has finally found his place. The night is a perfect mix of old memories and new beginnings, marked by laughter that heals and connections that have grown stronger. And with that,— not with a grand gesture or sweeping statement, but with a simple, joyful moment between friends, finally free of the weight they once carried, and ready for whatever comes next.

The sky is clear, dotted with stars that seem to glow brighter in the crisp night air. They stand side by side, watching their breath puff in the cool breeze, each lost in their own thoughts for a moment.

Jack glances over at Sophie, who has her arms crossed, looking up at the stars. "It's hard to believe, isn't it? That I've made it here."

Sophie smiles softly, still gazing at the sky. "Yeah… There were times I didn't think you would."

Jack nods, a content sigh escaping him. "And we've still got a long way to go." They share a knowing look, one filled with the quiet understanding that life will keep moving forward, and they're ready to move with it. The night feels peaceful, not bittersweet, as if the universe itself is giving them permission to move on—carrying their friends in their hearts, but no longer letting the weight of loss hold them down. Jack and Sophie exchange a smile, knowing that they have finally found a place where both the past and the future can coexist. There is peace. There is hope. And there is life—waiting for them to live it fully. The stars twinkle above, but Jack and Sophie no longer need to look to the sky for signs. Liam and Emily are with them always, as partners, as memories that have woven themselves into the fabric of who they've become. And they are ready, at last, to let themselves live. Life after-all is a path full of turns and twists.

In the shadows of winter, the world feels still,
A whisper of laughter, a haunting chill.
You're the ghost in my memory, a flickering light,
A promise of joy, now hidden from sight.

Each morning I rise, but the warmth feels far,
Your smile lingers, like a distant star.
Yet here I stand, a shadow of me,
Caught in a battle, struggling to be.

The weight of your absence, a heavy shroud,
I wear it like armor, though it drags me down.
I seek the laughter in children's embrace,
Finding comfort in their innocence, their grace.

But nights are the hardest, the silence so loud,
My heart, a wild bird, trapped in a cloud.
Dreams turn to nightmares, your face fades to gray,
How do I live in a world that's lost its way?

Yet, I know you'd want me to carry on,
To find the beauty in life, to sing a new song.
So I gather my courage, and with each step I take,
I hold on to love, for our shared heart's sake.

I sit with the sun as it fades into night,
Each moment, a choice, to grieve or to fight.
The past wraps around me, a bittersweet thread,
A tapestry woven with words left unsaid.

You taught me to love fiercely, to dance in the rain,
But here in the silence, I'm lost in the pain.
The echoes of laughter, the warmth of your hand,
Are treasures I carry, though hard to withstand.

I see your face in the smiles of the young,
In the hopes of tomorrow, our anthem unsung.
I fight for their futures, I carry your name,
Through struggles and triumphs, through joy and through pain.

So, I walk through the shadows, the heartache, the strife,
With a flicker of courage, igniting my life.
Each tear tells a story, each smile a start,
A testament of love, forever in my heart.

With every sunrise, I gather my strength,
Though grief is a river that runs wide in length.
It pulls me beneath, in its currents I fight,
Yet somehow, I rise to greet the new light.

The children I nurture, their laughter a balm,
In their joy, I find pieces of moments, so calm.
Through struggles and stories, through heartache and strife,
I see the reflections of a once vibrant life.

Yet still, in the quiet, your absence resounds,
A bittersweet echo that forever surrounds.
But in this journey, I learn to embrace,
The lessons of love that time cannot erase.

For as I heal, I see what you've left,
A legacy forged in love, not in regret.
So I turn to the future, with hope in my chest,
Carrying your spirit as I seek out the rest.

Together we tread on this winding road,
Two souls intertwined, bearing grief's heavy load.
Yet laughter breaks through the fog of despair,
In moments we cherish, in memories we share.

You hold my hand, through the dark and the light,
Reminding me gently that we're still in this fight.
In the warmth of your laughter, I find my way back,
To the joy we once savored, though time has turned black.

We wander through shadows, yet feel the sun's kiss,
In the spaces between us, we find our own bliss.
With every step forward, the weight lifts a bit,
And slowly, we learn to embrace what we've missed.

For love doesn't fade, it transforms, it grows,
Through trials and heartaches, the heart truly knows.
We'll carry our losses, our scars will remain,
But in love's gentle presence, we'll dance through the pain.

In the quietest moments, your voice fills the air,
A melody of comfort, a promise laid bare.
Through heartaches and memories, your spirit still glows,
A testament to love that forever bestows.

With each passing season, I learn to let go,
Of the sorrow that binds me, of the tears that flow.
For love is a garden, tended with care,
And in every new bloom, your essence is there.

So here's to the laughter, the struggles we face,
To the bonds that we cherish, to time and its grace.
As we navigate life, through the joy and the strife,
We honor your memory by embracing this life.

And in the reflection of those we've held dear,
We find our own strength, we shed every fear.
For love is the legacy, the gift we must share,
In the hearts of the living, your spirit is there.

Thank You ,
SEE YOU SOON.
Take Care!

(childeye)

My current address to meet or write to:

Childeye room, Nighoj, 414306

Mail - ichildeye@gmail.com

www.ingramcontent.com/pod-product-compliance
Lightning Source LLC
Chambersburg PA
CBHW062108160726
48282CB00026B/717
9788198124678